THE COMPLICATED MEDICAL
PATIENT

THE COMPLICATED MEDICAL PATIENT
New Approaches to Psychomedical Syndromes

John I. Walker, M.D.
*Department of Psychiatry
University of Texas
Health Science Center
San Antonio, Texas*

James Trig Brown, M.D.
and
Harry A. Gallis, M.D.
*Department of Medicine
Duke University Medical Center
Durham, North Carolina*

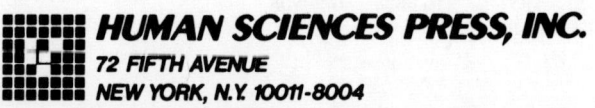

HUMAN SCIENCES PRESS, INC.
72 FIFTH AVENUE
NEW YORK, N.Y. 10011-8004

Copyright © 1987 by Human Sciences Press, Inc.
72 Fifth Avenue, New York, New York 10011

All rights reserved. No part of this work may be reproduced or utilized in any form or by any means, electronic or mechanical, including photocopying, microfilm and recording, or by any information storage and retrieval system without permission in writing from the publisher.

Printed in the United States of America
987654321

Library of Congress Cataloging-in-Publication Data

The Complicated medical patient.

  Includes bibliographies and index.
  1. Medicine, Psychosomatic. I. Walker, J. Ingram (John Ingram), 1944–   . II. Brown, J. Trig (James Trig) III. Gallis, Harry A. [DNLM: 1. Psychophysiologic Disorders. WM 90 C737]
RC49.C57   1987   616.08   86-20808
ISBN 0-89885-331-1

CONTENTS

Preface   9

Contributors   11

PART I. EATING AND METABOLIC DISORDERS   15

   1. **Anorexia Nervosa**   17
      W. J. Kenneth Rockwell, M.D.

   2. **Bulimia: Diagnostic and Therapeutic Considerations**   28
      Robert T. Harris, M.D.

PART II. PAIN SYNDROMES — 39

3. Management of Premenstrual Syndrome — 41
John F. Steege, M.D.
Anna L. Stout, Ph.D.
Sharon L. Rupp, R.N.C.

4. Fibromyalgia: A Disorder for all Physicians — 58
John R. Rice, M.D.

5. Headaches — 71
E. Wayne Massey, M.D.

6. Temporo Mandibular Joint Disorders: Diagnosis and Treatment — 90
Edward A. Dolan, D.D.S.

7. Irritable Bowel Syndrome — 120
Michael E. McLeod, M.D.

8. Perineal Pain: Prostatodynia or Prostatitis? — 131
Culley C. Carson III, M.D.

9. The Chronic Pain Patient: Behavioral Treatment Strategies — 138
John S. Jordan, Ph.D.
Francis J. Keefe, Ph.D.

PART III. SPELLS — 159

10. Seizures and Pseudoseizures — 161
J. Scott Luther, M.D.

11. Panic Attacks — 174
J. Trig Brown, M.D.

PART IV.		FACTITIAL DISEASES	185
	12.	Psychocutaneous Syndromes *Claude S. Burton, M.D.*	187
	13.	Factitial Fever *Harry A. Gallis, M.D.*	202
PART V.		PSYCHOSOMATIC MEDICINE REVISITED	211
	14.	Excessive Somatic Concern: Diagnostic and Treatment Issues *J. Trig Brown, M.D.* *John I. Walker, M.D.*	213
	15.	Depression in the Medical Patient *Gail Lynn Shaw, M.D.* *John I. Walker, M.D.*	231
	16.	The Medical Evaluation of Psychiatric Disease *Ann Weisler Edmundson, M.D.*	256
	17.	The Ill Physician: A Complicated Medical Patient *Conrad Fulkerson, M.D.*	270

Index *283*

PREFACE

Practitioners see complicated medical patients daily. The level of complexity depends not only on the patient and the patient's problem, but also on the physician's own training, experience, and practice style. In our experience the "complicated medical patient" is often that patient whose clinical picture is not easily reduced to biomedical solutions. These patients cannot be evaluated nor treated in a void; their behavior, family, and psychological development also must be examined to better understand their illnesses.

We use the term "psychomedical" disorders and avoid the term "psychosomatic" intentionally because of the variety of meanings subsumed by the latter term. Time has distilled Franz Alexander's traditional concept of psychosomatic disorders into the "magnificent seven": peptic ulcer, colitis, asthma, hypertension, neurodermatitis, arthritis, and thyrotoxicosis.[1] These seven are noticeably absent from this volume, a reflection of how the thinking in psychomedical syndromes is evolving.

Interestingly, if one examines Alexander's original text, his concept of psychosomatic disorders more closely resembles this current undertaking.[2] Anorexia nervosa, bulimia, nervous vomiting, esophageal spasms, chronic diarrhea, spastic colitis, chronic constipation, tachycardia, vasodepressor syncope, dermatitis factitia, fatigue states, and disorders of carbohydrate metabolism all share equal billing with the traditional seven. Why then did only seven of his syndromes survive to carry the label psychosomatic? It may be that these other disorders were recognized even then by his readers as complicated and hence the excellent clinical descriptions he gave them atrophied through the years.

This current work reviews the epidemiology, the clinical manifestations, and the medical evaluation needed when attending these patients. Our first goal is for the reader to become more comfortable in treating the syndromes described. The hope then is that these patients will begin to seem less complicated and our understanding of these complex problems will advance.

John I. Walker
J. Trig Brown
Harry A. Gallis

REFERENCES

1. Alexander F: The psychosomatic approach in medical therapy. In *The Scope of Psychoanalysis.* New York; Basic Books, 1961, pp. 345–358.
2. Alexander F: *Psychosomatic Medicine: Its Principles and Applications.* New York; W.W. Norton, 1950.

CONTRIBUTORS

James Trig Brown, M.D., Assistant Professor of Medicine, Duke University Medical Center, Durham, North Carolina.

Claude S. Burton, M.D., Associate in Medicine, Division of Dermatology, Duke University Medical Center, Durham, North Carolina.

Culley C. Carson III, M.D., Associate Professor of Urology, Duke University Medical Center, Durham, North Carolina.

Edward A. Dolan, D.D.S., Assistant Professor, Division of Oral and Maxillo-facial Surgery, Duke University Medical Center, Durham, North Carolina.

Ann Weisler Edmundson, M.D., Department of General Medicine, Duke University Medical Center, Durham, North Carolina; Department of Internal Medicine, University of Alabama at Birmingham, Montgomery Program.

CONTRIBUTORS

Conrad Fulkerson, M.D., Clinical Assistant Professor, Division of Psychosomatic Medicine, Department of Psychiatry, Duke University Medical Center, Durham, North Carolina.

Harry A. Gallis, M.D., Associate Professor of Medicine, Department of Medicine, Duke Medical Center, Durham, North Carolina.

Robert T. Harris, M.D., Associate in Medicine, Division of General Medicine, Department of Medicine, Duke University Medical Center, Durham, North Carolina.

John S. Jordan, PH.D., Assistant Professor of Medical Psychology, Department of Psychiatry, Duke University Medical Center, Durham, North Carolina.

Francis J. Keefe, Ph.D., Associate Professor of Medical Psychology, Department of Psychiatry, Duke University Medical Center, Durham, North Carolina.

J. Scott Luther, M.D., Assistant Professor of Medicine/Neurology, University of Texas Health Science Center, San Antonio, Texas.

E. Wayne Massey, M.D., Associate Professor of Medicine, Division of Neurology, Duke University Medical Center, Durham, North Carolina.

Michael E. McLeod, M.D., Professor of Medicine, Duke University Medical Center, Durham, North Carolina.

John R. Rice, M.D., Assistant Professor of Medicine, Division of Rheumatology and Immunology, Department of Medicine, Duke University School of Medicine, Durham, North Carolina.

W.J. Kenneth Rockwell, M.D., Director, Anorexia Nervosa/Bulimia Treatment Program and Assistant Professor of Psychiatry, Duke University Medical Center, Durham, North Carolina.

Sharon L. Rupp, R.N.C., Associate, Department of Obstetrics and Gynecology; Clinic Coordinator, Premenstrual Syndrome Clinic, Duke University Medical Center, Durham, North Carolina.

Gail Lynn Shaw, M.D., Duke University Medical Center, Durham, North Carolina.

John F. Steege, M.D., Assistant Professor, Department of Obstetrics and Gynecology, Co-Director, Premenstrual Syndrome Clinic, Duke University Medical Center, Durham, North Carolina.

Anna L. Stout, Ph.D., Assistant Professor, Division of Medical Psychology, Department of Psychiatry, Department of Obstetrics and Gynecology; Co-Director, Premenstrual Syndrome Clinic, Duke University Medical Center, Durham, North Carolina.

John I. Walker, M.D., Clinical Professor of Psychiatry, University of Texas, Health Science Center, San Antonio, Texas; Medical Director, Hill Country Hospital, Live Oak, Texas.

Part I

EATING AND METABOLIC DISORDERS

Chapter 1

ANOREXIA NERVOSA

W. J. Kenneth Rockwell, M.D.

Epidemiology and Diagnosis

Nowadays the term "Eating Disorders" refers to Anorexia Nervosa, Bulimia, and Atypical Eating Disorder, entities listed in the *Third Diagnostic and Statistical Manual of the American Psychiatric Association (DSM-III)*[1]. Whereas anorexia nervosa was named in 1874 and has been continuously discussed in the medical literature since then, bulimia, which denotes oxlike eating, did not appear as a diagnostic entity until recently. Although we have no old epidemiological studies on which to base comparisons, current belief is that there is a true increase in the incidence and prevalence in eating disorders in the United States and Western Europe. Approximately 95 percent of the victims of eating disorders are women, and in the adolescent and young adult female population the incidence of anorexia nervosa may be as high as 1 percent and that of bulimia 5 percent. Consequently, these illnesses can no longer be considered rare, particularly among young females.

The DSM-III diagnostic criteria for Anorexia Nervosa are as follows: A) Intense fear of becoming obese, which does not diminish as weight loss progresses; B) Disturbance of body image, e.g., claiming to "feel fat" even when emaciated; C) Weight loss of at least 25 percent of original body weight or, if under eighteen years of age, weight loss from original body weight plus projected weight gain expected from growth charts may be combined to make the 25 percent; D) Refusal to maintain body weight over a minimal normal weight for age and height; E) No known physical illness that would account for the weight loss. Bulimia will be dealt with in the next chapter.

Frequently accompanying the disordered eating behavior is the concomitant use and abuse of laxatives, diuretics, and stimulants such as diet pills and caffeine. The use of ipecac as an emetic is less frequent, but it is very dangerous in that it has been known to cause fatal emetine myocardiopathy. The abuse of any of the foregoing agents may be dangerous, and their use should be inquired about routinely during the course of a workup for an eating disorder. The physical complications of anorexia nervosa are essentially those of malnutrition and include: death by starvation, electrolyte depletion, cardiac arrhythmias, weakness and fatigue, famine edema, amenorrhea, dry skin, brittle nails, loss of hair, keratinemia, low serum protein and albumin, low red and white blood cell counts, low blood sugar, and constipation. Specific vitamin deficiencies are surprisingly rare, but are not unknown in this illness.

Before a diagnosis of anorexia nervosa has become firmly established, differentiating it from a variety of medical and psychiatric illnesses may be difficult. One is obliged to examine and test for specific illnesses not only because of mimicry but because anorexia nervosa often coexists with other illnesses. The endocrinological, gastrointestinal, and central nervous systems always require medical consideration, if not complete evaluation. The psychiatric differential includes depression, schizophrenia, and personality disorders with hysterical manifestations. Arriving reluctantly at a diagnosis of anorexia nervosa through exclusion of all other possibilities by exhaustive workups need not nor should not be done, as too much time is lost. The very distinct positive criteria on which to base a diagnosis are the overwhelming fear of fatness, the relentless pursuit of thinness, and the body image disturbance. In other words, the diagnosis is supported when the patient reports being too fat at the present, or that she would be too fat if she were 5 pounds heavier, when all other observers agree that the patient is much too thin. Since this body image disturbance occurs in some nonanorexic (including normal) people, it is not pathognomonic of the illness; nevertheless, the distorted body image attitude is virtually ubiquitous among anorexic patients.

Anorexia nervosa is the most lethal of psychiatric illnesses, with a mortality rate of between 5 and 10 percent. In a compilation of 16 studies in which a total of 737 patients had been followed for 2 or more years posttreatment, the mortality rate was 6.2 percent[2]. In the longest follow-up study to date, which included 94 patients, a few of whom had had the illness for 50 years or more, the mortality rate was 19.2 percent[3]. On the other hand, it is well known that individuals have recovered with very little or no treatment, either medical or psychiatric, although it is impossible to know what percentage of the total number such people represent. The prognosis is difficult to define because anorexia nervosa has a very wide range of severity. Factors that have been associated with poor outcome include: 1) long duration of illness; 2) older age of onset; 3) occurrence of bulimia and/or laxative abuse; 4) very low weight on admission; and 5) overestimation of own body size (3). It would seem that later age of onset is a contradictory finding in that older individuals would presumably have developed more independence and a greater sense of identity—features found lacking in the psychological makeup of sick anorexics. Although the data are yet to be developed, one might suppose that individuals with older onset have an occult history of dietary disturbances or have been able to sustain a premorbid disposition for the illness for a greater period of time. In any event, it is now generally accepted clinical wisdom that the earlier the illness is detected and the sooner treatment begins, the better is the outlook.

Early signs of illness include:

1. *Cessation of menses.* In between one-fourth and one-third of patients, menses become disturbed or cease prior to the onset

of weight loss. However, in some of these patients a careful history will reveal that disturbed eating patterns or even dietary chaos have already commenced.
2. *Change in eating habits.* This may come about in a variety of ways, including a physician-prescribed diet for weight loss purposes; or the patient herself may initiate a diet because her friends are doing it "just to lose a few pounds." Such dieting is extremely common and implies nothing initially. A change in goal weight downward to more than a few pounds below that initially set is a warning sign. Crash, fad, and unbalanced diets should be advised against in any event; but anorexics are more likely to prescribe for themselves and consistently and rigidly exclude fats and carbohydrates than are other dieters. Surreptitious dieting, if it can be detected, is always a danger signal, as is a prolonged shift to solitary eating.
3. *The development of an attitudinal and behavioral preoccupation with food, weight, and eating.*
4. *Concomitantly related behaviors such as an increase in exercise related activities to inexplicably high levels and withdrawal from social relationships.*

Etiology

The etiology of anorexia nervosa is unknown but is probably multidetermined. A number of predisposing factors have been found in association with anorexia nervosa. The age and sex distribution are well known; this is a disease of primarily adolescent and young adult females. The illness is found in all social classes but with the preponderance in upper and middle classes. The family ethos of anorexic girls appears to magnify our cultural emphasis on thinness, fitness, and high mental and physical performance. Parents of anorexics are likely to be older than average and are more likely to have a history of affective illness. Anorexia nervosa in siblings occurs more often than by chance, and although in the relatively small number of twin pairs studied so far the concordance for monozygotic twins is 50 percent and for dizygotic twins 10 percent, this difference can be as well accounted for at the present time on a psychological basis as on a genetic one. The specific interactions of parents with their anorexic child appear to give rise to difficulties in separation and autonomy on the part of the child, but it is difficult to separate cause and effect in studying these interactions. Nevertheless, individuals with anorexia nervosa always demonstrate difficulties in autonomy and identity with separation concerns and fears of becoming an adult with what that implies in terms of emotional independence, active sexuality, and the responsibilities of being a parent. Anorexics may also have a difficulty in awareness of or interpretation of their internal stimuli, specifically those related to hunger and satiety. A disproportionate number give a history of overweight in childhood or of weight instability. Maintaining the concrete thought processes of latency-age childhood rather than developing the abstract mode of thinking during adolescence may represent a basic cognitive factor predisposing to anorexia nervosa. Evidence for a biological factor basic to the etiology of anorexia is now lacking, but a primary hypothalamic disorder, the influence of a peptide or some other neurohumor, or even contribution from a peripheral defect have not been ruled out.

Treatment

No single treatment or combination of treatments has been found that will consistently ameliorate anorexia nervosa. A multimodel approach can be used rationally and is indicated, even though occasionally one modality will suffice. As with other illnesses, the hospital should be used only when necessary. With earlier detection and the availability of more therapists familiar with anorexia, the need for extensive hospitalizations should diminish. The need for hospitalization is based on clinical judgment and the criteria to be considered usually include the following: weight loss, failure of outpatient treatment, severe metabolic abnormality, and psychic status. Weight loss to below 60 percent of ideal body weight is, alone, an indication for hospitalization. Often enough weight loss of 20 to 25 percent below ideal body weight in conjunction with other factors will prompt hospitalization. Failure of outpatient treatment that has been consistent and continuous for 6 or more months should raise a question of hospitalization or a change in the method of outpatient treatment. With respect to metabolic abnormality, a serum potassium below 2.0 mEq/L is sufficient reason for hospitalization as are repeated K+ levels below 2.5 mEq/L. Such metabolic abnormalities are usually associated with vomiting or laxative or diuretic abuse, but they can be achieved by severe food restriction. Severe dysphoria with depression or anxiety, usually due to conflict with parents or spouse, may require at least brief hospitalization to bring the conflict under control. Depending on its extent and intensity, suicidal ideation would be an indication for hospitalization in any event, but since approximately one-third of the mortality associated with anorexia nervosa is due to suicide, this possibility must always be evaluated.

In-hospital treatment has two major objectives, approached simultaneously, but with the emphasis shifting from one to the other as the hospitalization progresses. These are 1) physiological and 2) psychosocial restitution. Physiological restitution is given first consideration because it is felt to be necessary for the work of psychosocial rehabilitation to proceed efficiently, if at all. Physiological restitution consists of "nutritional rehabilitation" with weight restoration and stabilization, and the cessation of behaviors concomitant with eating disorders, such as use of laxatives, diuretics, diet pills, or emetics. All of these objectives can be accomplished while in hospital. Psychosocial restitution consists of 1) assuming responsibility for eating and related behaviors and weight control; 2) reducing intensity of obsessive focus on eating, weight and body image; 3) broadening range of activities and interests; 4) examining family relationships, effecting disentanglements, and establishing self-boundary within the family; 5) examining peer relationships and effecting age-appropriate socialization processes; and 6) assuming responsibility for own feelings and behaviors and establishing self-boundary in relation to all others. In hospitals, the first of these can be accomplished, but only a beginning can be made in accomplishing the last five.

The components of an in-hospital treatment program are listed in Table 1-1. Since a treatise on treatment is beyond the scope of this chapter, a few comments must suffice. An activities

Table 1-1. Components of an In-Hospital Treatment Program for Anorexia Nervosa (Listed Alphabetically)

1. ACTIVITIES PROGRAM
    Art Therapy
    Athletics
    Exercise
    Occupational Therapy
    School
    Therapeutic Movement Group
2. BEHAVIOR MODIFICATION
    "High" Structure
    "Low" Structure
3. DIETETIC CONSULTATION AND EDUCATION
4. FAMILY THERAPY
5. HOSPITAL MILIEU
6. MEDICATION
    Antidepressants
    Anxiolytics
    Appetite/Weight Related
7. NURSING CARE
8. PSYCHOPHYSIOLOGIC: BIOFEEDBACK
9. PSYCHOTHERAPY
    Group
    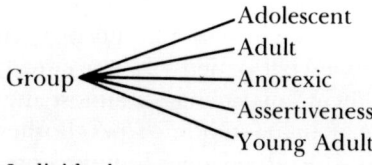
    - Adolescent
    - Adult
    - Anorexic
    - Assertiveness
    - Young Adult
    Individual
10. SELF-HELP GROUP
    Designated Patient
    Family
    Parents

program can be useful in more directions than just giving patients a way to pass the time. It can help them reduce their obsessive focus on food and weight and can enhance their sense of achievement and identity. Behavior modification as the sole modality used to promote weight gain is contraindicated. The use of externally provided structure with its accompanying loss of self-determined activity (implied in the need for hospitalization in the first place) is often necessary to accomplish any weight gain whatsoever. A variety of "rewards" (privileges) and "punishments" (restrictions) can be elaborated in conjunction with each individual's needs and desires that will provide the necessary support and structure. Occasionally a great number of restrictions and privileges must be developed to conform to an equally large number of contingencies presented by the patient: hence the need for "high structure" behavior modification.

The dietitian consults with patients on their day-to-day menus and with the dietary service on their implementation. The regulation of balanced nutrition, normal eating patterns, and numbers of calories to provide weight gain or maintenance are calculated and not left to chance. Furthermore, although anorexics are correctly known to be masters at calorie counting, many lack basic knowledge of proper nutrition. Evaluation of the patient's parents, and spouse if she is married, is routine if they are available. Other family members may also enter the picture. At least several sessions with family members or spouse are useful and more often than not extended family or marital therapy is indicated. Following this, couples therapy for the parents or individual therapy for one or both parents or spouse is often recommended. For adolescent patients who are living at home, family therapy, often including siblings, is almost always needed and will often be the primary mode of psychotherapy. This should be commenced while the patient is in the hospital, if possible. The effect of the hospital milieu on treatment of the anorexic has not been well studied, but important factors to consider are whether the unit is medical, psychiatric, or pediatric, whether locked or unlocked, and what types of patients it includes.

At the present time medication is an adjunct to therapy. There is no medication that has been consistently useful in helping to promote weight gain or maintain it in patients with anorexia nervosa. The full range of psychoactive medications has been tried, as well as some additional compounds that influence appetite and weight control. Some anorexics have had their depressions relieved by treatment with antidepressants but without any significant effect on their anorexic processes or the related weight problems. Antidepressants and anxiolytics are used empirically, with more or less success, for relief of depression and anxiety.

Nursing care provides the foundation for and day-to-day implementation of both the physiological and psychosocial objectives of in-hospital treatment. The quality of the program is directly related to the quality of the nursing care and does not exceed it. A psychophysiologic treatment such as biofeedback can be a useful adjunct to treatment in that it may enable the patient to gain a greater sense of control and mastery over her body by means that are unrelated to food and weight. In addition to family therapy, group and individual psychotherapy are basic modalities for helping to implement the psychosocial objectives. Individual, group, and family therapy are usually initiated simultaneously. Most of our anorexic patients have felt that they benefited from assertiveness training and from group therapy with other anorexic and eating-disordered patients. Therapy in age-appropriate groups that include noneating disordered patients is also useful, often initiated after experience in the other two types of groups and when the anorexic patient has broken out of her obsessive focus on food and is able to talk about problems that are not food and weight related. Self-help groups are primarily populated by outpatients and their families, but such a group can be well used by the family of an anorexic while she is in hospital, with a view to follow-up in the group by everyone after the patient is discharged. In particular, the parents of patients just entering treatment usually feel confused and isolated, states that are optimally dealt with in a well-conducted self-help group.

Outpatient therapy begins with an evaluation of the patient and her family or husband. Once again, for younger adolescents living at home, family therapy is often the treatment of choice and may be the sole modality needed. For older adolescents and adults, family therapy is often indicated for the initial phase of treatment and is then followed by individual psychotherapy for the patient and marital or individual therapy for her parents.

Likewise, couples therapy for the married patients is often followed by individual psychotherapy for one or both of the partners. Patients and their families may make use of self-help group organizations or other types of group experiences at the same time. Anorexic patients are notoriously reluctant to engage in treatment, but many will join a self-help group if it is available, and this should be encouraged. Dietetic consultation and education is helpful in the outpatient setting but dietitians should encourage their patients not to make this their sole professional contact. As a final stage of treatment, most anorexics will benefit from a period of individual psychotherapy that will help them consolidate their previous gains and achieve an even greater level of autonomy and independence.

The major change that has occurred in recent years with regard to the treatment of anorexia nervosa is that both the disordered physiology and eating behavior of the patient and the concomitant psychological disturbances are taken into account and dealt with simultaneously, the emphasis in treatment being placed where the derangement is greater. Such a dual focus usually requires a team approach employing a number of different interventions simultaneously and sequentially.

REFERENCES

1. *Diagnostic and Statistical Manual of Mental Disorders*, 3rd ed, Washington DC, American Psychiatric Association, 1980.
2. Hsu LKG: Outcome of anorexia nervosa: A review of the literature (1954–1978). *Arch Gen Psychiatry* 1980; 9:1041–1046.
3. Theander S: Research on outcome and prognosis of anorexia nervosa and some results from a Swedish long-term study. *Int J Eating Disorders* 1983; 2(4):167–174.

BIBLIOGRAPHY

Andersen AE: *Practical Comprehensive Treatment of Anorexia Nervosa and Bulimia*. Baltimore, Johns Hopkins University Press, 1985.
Bruch, H: *Eating Disorders: Obesity, Anorexia Nervosa, and the Person Within*. New York, Basic Books, 1973.

Bruch, H: *The Golden Cage: The Enigma of Anorexia Nervosa.* Cambridge, MA, Harvard University Press, 1978.

Garfinkel PE, Garner DM: *Anorexia Nervosa: A Multidimensional Perspective* New York, Brunner/Mazel, 1982.

Garner DM, Garfinkel PE (Eds(Eds): *Handbook of Psychotherapy for Anorexia Nervosa and Bulimia.* New York, Guilford Press, 1985.

Larocca FEF (Ed): *Eating Disorders: Effective Care and Treatment* (Vol. I.). St. Louis, Ishiyaku EuroAmerica, 1985.

Chapter 2

BULIMIA

Diagnostic and Therapeutic Considerations

Robert T. Harris, M.D.

Bulimia, known also as bulimia nervosa and bulimarexia, is characterized by the self-perpetuating practice of binge eating followed by self-induced vomiting or other forms of purging. Though less studied and only recognized as a distinct eating disorder in the 1980s, bulimia is likely the most common. As in anorexia nervosa, it is most frequent among young, white females. Population surveys have generally been limited to college campuses where 19 percent of the females and 5 percent of the males are reported to fulfill (DSM-III, 1980) criteria for bulimia[1]. A nonstudent group of 300 suburban shoppers reported on questionnaires a 0.7 percent history of anorexia nervosa and a 10.3 percent history of bulimia, using DSM-III criteria, with the greatest frequency of bulimia in women between thirteen and thirty years of age[2].

Bulimia was previously thought to be a "burned out" form of anorexia nervosa, since Russell found a history of anorexia nervosa in 50 percent of the bulimic women he studied[3]. A more recent report, however, found a history of anorexia nervosa in only 5 percent of 509 bulimic women interviewed, thus underscoring it as a distinct disorder[4].

Making the Diagnosis of Bulimia

The diagnostic criteria are shown in Table 2-1. Binge eating is done in secrecy and is not in response to the physiologic sense of hunger. Foods eaten are easily ingested with little chewing and are highly caloric. Assorted foods containing 20,000 calories or more may be consumed in an hour. Commonly, patients report eating a half-gallon of ice cream or a whole cake or bag of cookies in less than an hour.

Binges are usually in response to psychosocial stresses that may or may not be recognized by the patient. During binges some patients report "automatic" behavior with a sense of depersonalization and feelings of separation from the environment. Binges stop with self-induced vomiting, abdominal discomfort, social interruption, abuse of cathartic or diuretic drugs, or fatigue and sleep. Self-induced vomiting is interspersed between periods

Table 2-1. Bulimia: Diagnostic Criteria—Adapted from Diagnostic and Statistical Manual of Mental Disorders, 3rd Edition

A. Recurrent episodes of binge eating
B. At least three of the following:
　1) consumption of high-caloric, easily ingested food during a binge
　2) inconspicuous eating during a binge
　3) termination of such eating episodes by abdominal pain, sleep, social interruption, or self-induced vomiting
　4) repeated attempts to lose weight by severely restrictive diets, self-induced vomiting, or use of cathartics or diuretics
　5) frequent weight fluctuations greater than 10 pounds due to alternating binges and fasts
C. Awareness that the eating pattern is abnormal and fear of not being able to stop eating voluntarily.
D. Depressed mood and self-deprecating thoughts following eating binges.
E. The bulimic episodes are not due to anorexia nervosa or any known physical disorder.

of binge eating and the binge-purge cycle may continue for several hours. Most bulimic episodes occur at night but some patients report near control of their daily lives by bulimic episodes. Compromised job performance may be recognized by the patient or her employer.

A period of daily bulimic episodes may be followed by a return to a more normal eating pattern or by self-imposed starvation with modest weight loss. More self-induced vomiting, cathartic or diuretic drug use, or excessive exercise may accompany intentional starvation. Thus, depending on which behavior predominates at a given time, a bulimic patient's weight may vary considerably. Near-ideal body weight may be maintained for long periods, but 10 percent fluctuations above or below the usual weight are common. Therefore, bulimia is not diagnosable by the pound as is the case with anorexia nervosa.

Psychologically, bulimic patients are acutely aware of their abnormal eating behavior. They often share the "fear of fatness" seen in anorexic patients but they fear more the very behavior they exhibit—i.e., loss of control of eating. Self-induced vomiting, exercise, and purgative drug use are assumed to prevent weight gain anticipated from binge eating. Despite these "undoing" maneuvers, feelings of extreme guilt and shame often overwhelm the patient; self-deprecating thoughts and depression are common. Concurrent diagnoses of dysthymic disorder and major depression are reported in over 50 percent of bulimic patients[5].

With bulimia, the primary care physician is frequently in the critical role of making the diagnosis. The lack of overt physical signs (e.g. emaciation, as seen in anorexia nervosa) and the facts that bulimic individuals are usually near normal weight and typically practice their behavior in secrecy impede the diagnostic process.

When the physician's suspicion is raised that bulimia may underlie a patient's visit, a series of questions may be helpful in making a diagnosis. The interview should begin with open-ended, nonthreatening questions and move, guided by the patient's answers, to more specific inquiries. Examples follow.

Open-ended questions:

1. How has your weight been recently? Does it change rapidly, up and down?

2. Are you happy with your weight and appearance?
3. How has your appetite been recently?
4. What is your typical day's diet like?
5. How has your mood been recently? Does eating cause your feelings to change, for the better or worse?

Directed questions:

1. Are there certain foods that give you trouble or that you might eat in excess if you feel sad, angry, or nervous?
2. Do you ever fear that you might eat more than you should or that you might not be able to stop eating?
3. Does overeating cause you to feel guilty or depressed?
4. What do you do in response to those guilt feelings you have when you overeat (self-induced vomiting, exercise, laxatives)?
5. Are you more likely to overeat in private or with others around?
6. Have you discussed your concerns about overeating or your body-weight and appearance with anyone?

CLINICAL FINDINGS AND COMPLICATIONS

Medical complications may also bring the bulimic patient to the primary physician[6]. There are no classic physical findings in bulimia as in anorexia nervosa (emaciation, lanugo, hypotension); clinical findings are reflective of complications of the various aberrant behaviors (see Table 2-2).

Bulimic patients may occasionally self-impose starvation, though it is typically of short duration and results in modest weight loss. The hazards of intentional malnourishment in bulimia, should it be prolonged, are the same as those seen in anorexia nervosa.

Binge eating that ends a period of self-imposed starvation may carry greater risk for complications than binge eating interjected into a more normal eating pattern. Acute gastric dilatation is a hazard in this setting just as in the refeeding of anorexic patients. The dilatation is out of proportion to that expected from simply ingesting a large volume of food and suggests a gastric neurogenic disturbance[7]. Severe abdominal pain

Table 2-2. Bulimia: Clinical Findings and Complications

Organ System	Intentional Malnourishment	Binge Eating	Self-Induced Vomiting	Cathartic Abuse	Diuretic Abuse
Endocrine/metabolic	Amenorrhea; Infertility	—	—	—	—
Cardiovascular/pulmonary	Heart failure; bradycardia	Heart failure; refeeding edema; ? hypertension	Aspiration pneumonitis	Myocarditis (from impecac abuse); hypokalemic cardiomyopathy; volume loss	—
Renal/electrolyte disorders	Reduced glomerular filtration rate; tubular dysfunction	—	Metabolic alkalosis; hypokalemia	Hypokalemia; kaliopenic nephropathy	Hypokalemia; hyponatremia

Hematologic	Anemia; leukopenia; thrombocytopenia	—	—	—
Alimentary tract	Constipation; hemorrhoid exacerbation; delayed gastric emptying	Gastric dilatation or rupture; pancreatitis; liver enzymes increased	Oral cavity trauma; tooth enamel erosion; esophagitis; Mallory-Weiss syndrome; esophageal rupture; parotid enlargement	Hypokalemic ileus; melanosis coli; cathartic colon
Neurologic/psychiatric	Depression; hypothermia; lack of rapid eye movement sleep	Guilt feelings	—	—

and distention, nausea and vomiting may occur. Marked hypovolemia and hypochloremic metabolic alkalosis often accompany dilatation. The severest cases involve gastric rupture which carries a high mortality rate. Other gastrointestinal complications of binge eating include postbinge pancreatitis[8] and transient elevations in liver enzymes. Heart failure is a potential hazard in the binge eating patient who has previously starved herself just as in the anorexic patient being refed. Binge eating of high caloric, high salt-containing foods on a regular basis may accelerate the development of hypertension and early atherosclerosis.

Self-induced vomiting, with a frequency reported as high as 35 to 40 times a day threatens the bulimic patient with esophagitis and Mallory-Weiss tears[3]. A medical emergency is created by esophageal rupture which may result from prolonged vomiting. The frequent presence of acidic vomitus in the oral cavity accounts for the erosion of dental enamel in bulimic patients[9]. Painless bilateral parotid enlargement also is likely a result of frequent vomiting and may serve as a physical exam marker of recent bulimic behavior[10]. Aspiration pneumonitis is a potential pulmonary hazard of vomiting which may present as adult respiratory distress syndrome in its severest form. Hypokalemic metabolic alkalosis also may result from frequent vomiting, with hypokalemia triggering dangerous arrhythmias.

Cathartic drug abuse by bulimic patients includes the abuse of emetic agents and laxatives. Occasionally used by bulimics to invoke vomiting, ipecac syrup is potentially harmful in that a fatal form of myocarditis has been described; patients may present with chest pain, arrhythmias, or heart failure. The bulimic laxative abuser assumes that a large stool volume will rid her of unwanted calories from preceding binges. A recent study has refuted this notion[11]. Weight loss may result, however, from the volume loss and dehydration that accompany laxative-induced diarrhea. Chronic laxative use changes normal stool electrolyte concentrations, promoting potassium losses. Hypokalemia is manifested by complaints of fatigability, muscle cramps or weakness, headache, palpitations, and abdominal pain. End-organ disturbances from hypokalemia include cardiomyopathy, life-threatening arrhythmias, nephropathy manifested by diminished urinary concentrating ability and adynamic paralytic ileus.

Abuse of stimulant laxatives can result in cathartic colon, wherein "the colon is converted into an inert tube incapable of conducting normal peristalsis . . . without the aid of large doses of laxatives"[12]. Melanosis coli is a benign discoloration of the colonic mucosa due to long-term use of anthraquinone-containing laxatives. Constipation, alone or alternating with diarrhea, is common in laxative abusers. Misinterpretation of delayed stools as constipation after catharsis from laxative action may trigger a repetitive physiologic-behavioral vicious cycle that perpetuates laxative abuse.

A similar physiologic-behavioral vicious cycle can be set in motion with diuretic abuse, occasionally practiced by bulimic patients as a presumed weight control maneuver. Hypokalemia from diuretic abuse can produce weakness, cramps, abdominal pain, polyuria, and constipation. The constipation can trigger the laxative abuse cycle. The polyuria typically produces polydipsia, a bloated feeling, and possible edema which may be misinterpreted as increased body fat thus perpetuating diuretic abuse.

TREATMENT

Once the diagnosis is established, involving the patient in treatment is usually not difficult, since most patients want help. Determining the most effective treatment is difficult, however, since no studies of long-term, well-designed treatment programs have been reported. Three components comprise the optimal treatment program:

1. correction of medical complications;
2. behavioral and psychotherapy;
3. pharmacotherapy.

Mandatory hospitalization is not indicated for the treatment of bulimia, since severe malnourishment is not usually a problem; but severe medical complications or profound depression may warrant hospitalization.

Behavioral therapy combined with psychotherapy appears

most beneficial as a definitive treatment. A three-stage, cognitive-behavioral technique has been reported by Fairburn to demonstrate short-term success[13]. Briefly, stage one involves establishing the abnormal behavioral pattern through self-monitoring and then developing an "eating pattern prescription" which specifies exact menus, situations, and times for meals. Alternative pleasurable activities are listed and are to be selected when tempted to binge and purge. Nutritional and medical counsel are also provided. Stage two introduces limited quantities of previously binged foods (e.g., ice cream) and focuses on developing problem-solving techniques and a healthier self-image. Stage three is the maintenance phase which supports progress and plans strategies for handling anticipated relapses.

Supportive psychotherapy is useful as definitive treatment begins, and this can be provided by the primary care physician. Insight-oriented psychotherapy (by the primary physician or a psychiatrist) is needed in cases of concurrent major depression. Enlisting family support through family interviews can be helpful when the patient feels comfortable revealing her problem to her family. Family therapy may also be needed.

Much interest has been generated in the use of antidepressant medication for bulimia treatment. The possible association between major depression and bulimia is supported by the following lines of evidence:

1. The lifetime incidence of major depression in bulimic patients is as high as 66 percent[14];
2. From one-half to two-thirds of tested bulimic patients have shown nonsuppression of plasma cortisol at 4 p.m. on the day following an 11 p.m. dose of 1 mg dexamethasone[14], i.e. positive results on the modified dexamethasone suppression test, is a biologic marker in about 50 percent of cases of major depression;
3. Nearly 50 percent of 33 bulimic patients had a first-degree relative with depression[15].

Imipramine was tested in a double-blind, placebo-controlled study among 19 bulimic women, all of whom met DSM-III criteria for bulimia[5]. Ten of the 19 patients also met DSM-III criteria for depression. The use of imipramine over 6 weeks resulted in a 70 percent reduction in frequency of bulimic episodes and a 50 percent reduction in Hamilton depression scale scores, both significant changes compared to placebo.

Large series, long-term clinical trials using tricyclic antidepressants have not been reported to date. Therefore, antidepressant medication can be recommended only in bulimic patients with clear-cut evidence of concurrent depression. Though antidepressant medication may prove beneficial in nondepressed patients as well, its use will likely remain adjunctive to the other behavioral and psychotherapeutic treatments described.

REFERENCES

1. Halmi KA, Falk JR, Schwartz E: Binge-eating and vomiting: A survey of a college population. *Psychol Med* 1981;11:697.
2. Pope HG, Hudson JI, Yurgelun-Todd D: Anorexia nervosa and bulimia among 300 suburban women shoppers. *Am J Psychiatry* 1984;141:292.
3. Russell GFM: Bulimia nervosa. *Psychol Med* 1979;9:429.
4. Johnson CL, Struckey MK, Lewis LD et al: A survey of 509 cases of self-reported bulimia. In Darby PL et al (Eds), *Anorexia Nervosa: Recent Developments in Research*. New York, Alan R. Liss, 1983.
5. Pope HG, Hudson JI, Jonas JM: Bulimia treated with imipramine: A placebo-controlled, double-blind study. *Am J Psychiatry* 1983;140:554.
6. Harris RT: Bulimarexia and related serious eating disorders with medical complications. *Ann Intern Med* 1983;99:800.
7. Scobie BA: Acute gastric dilatation and duodenal ileus in anorexia nervosa. *Med J Aust* 1973;2:932.
8. Gryboski J, Hillemeier C, Kocoshis S: Refeeding pancreatitis in malnourished children. *J Pediatr* 1980;97:441.
9. Hurst PS, Lacey JH, Crisp AH: Teeth, vomiting and diet: A study of the dental characteristics of seventeen anorexia nervosa patients. *Postgrad Med J* 1977;53:298.

10. Levin PA, Falko JM, Dixon K et al: Benign parotid enlargement in bulimia. *Ann Intern Med* 1980;93:827.
11. Bo-Linn GW, Santa Ana CA, Morawski SG et al: Purging and calorie absorption in bulimic patients and normal women. *Ann Intern Med* 1983;99:14.
12. Oster JR, Materson BJ, Rogers AI: Laxative abuse syndrome. *Am J Gastroenterol* 1980;74:451.
13. Fairburn CG: Bulimia: Its epidemiology and management. In Stunkard AJ, Stellar E (Eds), *Eating and Its Disorders*. New York, Raven Press, 1984.
14. Hudson JI, Pope HG, Jonas JM: Treatment of bulimia with antidepressants: Theoretical considerations and clinical findings. In Stunkard AJ, Stellar E (Eds), *Eating and Its Disorders*. New York, Raven Press, 1984.
15. Pyle RL, Mitchell JE, Eckert ED: Bulimia: A report of 34 cases. *J Clin Psychiatry* 1981;42:60.

Part II

PAIN SYNDROMES

Chapter 3

MANAGEMENT OF PREMENSTRUAL SYNDROME

John F. Steege, M.D.
Anna L. Stout, Ph.D.
Sharon L. Rupp, R.N.C.

Recently much attention has been given to an age-old problem: the changes that many women experience premenstrually. When these changes are more severe, they have been labeled "premenstrual syndrome" or "PMS." These pages will review definitions of PMS, self-help measures, and pharmacologic and counseling treatments.

PMS: The Problem

The impact of the menstrual cycle on the human body is profound. Although accurate incidence figures are difficult to obtain and vary with the definition of PMS, many women experience some negative feelings or physical and emotional change before the onset of menses. Many also experience positive feelings of increased energy, greater sensitivity both emotionally and artistically, and greater creativity for a week or two prior to the beginning of the menstrual flow. Approximately 65 well recognized medical diseases and 115 normal events in the body's physiologic makeup may be influenced by the menstrual cycle.

It is no wonder, then, that women who experience severe changes premenstrually may notice a wide variety of symptoms. Approximately 150 symptoms have been described at one time or another as being related to the menstrual cycle.[1]

The symptoms of PMS can be grouped as described in Table 3-1. Our experience tells us that women who experience more severe emotional changes premenstrually do not necessarily experience more severe physical changes. Rather, they find emotional changes extremely disturbing and disruptive in their personal relationships and their ability to function at work and home. This is consistent with Clare's[2] finding that women with psychiatric ill-health reported more psychiatric and behavioral premenstrual symptoms, although they did not differ from psychiatrically "healthy" women in their report of physical symptoms premenstrually.

A large number of etiologic theories have been proposed to explain premenstrual changes (Table 3-2). Although there is scanty direct evidence to support any one of these theories over another,[3] a growing number of investigators feel that physiologic "triggers" of premenstrual events will be discovered. An equally dedicated group has demonstrated to their own satisfaction that sociocultural conditioning, environmental stresses, conflict in relationships, and psychiatric illness and personality disorders can greatly augment premenstrual changes. Two experiments from the literature illustrate the differing perspectives. The first is the very ingenious experiment of Ruble et al.[4] in which undergraduate volunteers were told that a "brain wave test" could determine the phase of their menstrual cycle. When responding to a questionnaire about premenstrual symptoms, those students who were misled to believe that they were premenstrual rather than postovulatory, indeed reported a much higher level of premenstrual symptoms. This result certainly attests to the power of sociocultural influences and/or expectations upon the reporting of subjective symptoms. The second experiment is that performed by Irwin et al.[5] The investigator withdrew units of blood in the follicular and luteal phases from 12 women and later reinfused these same units into the donors under double-blind conditions. The cycle phases of approximately 90 percent of the units were identified correctly. The women were typically able to identify

Table 3-1. Common Symptoms of Premenstrual Syndrome*

Affective

  Sadness
  Anxiety
  Anger
  Irritability
  Labile mood

Pain

  Headaches
  Breast tenderness
  Joint and muscle pain

Autonomic

  Nausea
  Diarrhea
  Palpitations
  Sweating

Fluid

  Bloating
  Weight gain
  Decreased urination
  Swelling

Behavioral

  Decreased motivation
  Poor impulse control
  Decreased efficiency
  Social isolation

Cognitive

  Decreased concentration
  Indecision
  Paranoia
  Sensitive to rejection
  Suicidal ideation

Neurovegetative

  Insomnia
  Hypersomnia
  Anorexia
  Craving for certain foods
  Fatigue
  Lethargy
  Agitation
  Libido change

Central Nervous System

  Clumsiness
  Seizures
  Dizziness
  Vertigo
  Paresthesias
  Tremors

Dermatologiocal

  Acne
  Greasy hair
  Dry hair

*From Rubinow DR, Roy-Byrne, P: Premenstrual syndromes: Overview from a methodologic perspective. *Am J Psychiatry* 1984; 141(2):163–172.

Table 3-2. Proposed Etiologies for Premenstrual Syndrome

Ovarian hormonal

    Estrogen
    Progesterone

Fluid and electrolyte normonal

    Prolactin
    Aldosterone
    Renin/angiotensin
    Vasopressin

Other hormonal

    Endorphine/enkephalins
    a-melanocyte stimulating hormone
    Glucocorticoid
    Androgen
    Insulin
    Melatonin

Neurotransmitter

    Monoamines (5-hydroxytryptamine, norepinephrine, dopamine)
    Acetylcholine

Other

    Vitamin B_6/magnesium
    Psychological basis
    Prostaglandins

the premenstrual units by noticing feelings of irritability, depression, and fatigue within the first few hours following infusion of the premenstrually donated plasma. Although unconfirmed, this is tantalizing evidence that there may indeed by some biochemical triggers to premenstrual symptoms in some women.

Even with etiologic questions unsettled, this complex disorder deserves a most careful evaluation in order to accomplish the best treatment results.

Making the Diagnosis

Retrospective impressions of premenstrual symptoms are often confirmed by prospective recording. However, events are more easily recalled when paired, perhaps especially when the event is interpreted as physiologic, and it is paired to another more clearly physiologic event. For instance, if a migraine headache occurs during menstruation, it is more likely to be recalled than a migraine occurring at other times in the cycle.

For these reasons, most investigators have found it best to first inventory a woman's major symptoms and then have her chart those symptoms on a daily basis using one type of calendar or another. The degree of cyclicity can then be easily and more reliably determined. We employ the Premenstrual Assessment Form[6] due to its value as a research instrument and because its validity as a psychometric instrument has been more extensively tested.[1] We then ask patients to complete daily rating forms based on this questionnaire.

A thorough physical examination is needed to look for medical illnesses that may mimic PMS symptoms. For example, lower abdominal and pelvic cramping and aching may be caused by endometriosis, large fibroids, or adenomyosis. Screening blood chemistries and a thyroid panel are useful as well. Various hormone levels such as progesterone are useful in deciding whether the menstrual cycle is normal in certain ways, but none of them "diagnose" premenstrual syndrome.

PMS can occur at any age after menstruation has begun. However, women are often most severely affected during their thirties and forties. Although some clinicians have postulated that high parity, taking birth control pills, and the absence of dysmenorrhea are associated with PMS, most of these associations have not been confirmed. For example, there is no credible published evidence that taking birth control pills aggravates premenstrual symptoms with any regularity, nor that they make a person more likely to get severe PMS symptoms after discontinuing the pills. Some women with premenstrual depression may experience worsened symptoms on oral contraceptives, however.[7] Similarly, although some women will note the beginning of PMS symptoms after childbirth, the majority do not seem to follow that pattern, or any other pattern relating events in reproduction (sterilization, etc.) to the beginning of PMS symptoms. It has been said that menstrual cramps are seldom present in women with PMS.[8] Our experience[9] and that of others has been quite contrary to this, since we find that many women with more severe PMS also have more severe menstrual cramps.

Psychological assessment assists in the overall evaluation of the PMS sufferer. In a population of 100 women referred for PMS evaluation, 64 percent had clinically elevated Minnesota Multiphasic Personality Inventory (MMPI) profiles when these tests were completed in the follicular phase (Table 3-3).[10] Keye et al.[11] have shown that these profiles worsen in the luteal phase. A standardized depression inventory such as the Beck Depression Inventory[12] or the Hamilton Depression Scale completed in the follicular and luteal phases of the cycle will help distinguish between continuous and premenstrual depression. Finally, we employ an unstructured psychological interview to evaluate general psychiatric status and screening questionnaires and an interview

Table 3-3. Classification of Minnesota Multiphasic Personality Inventory (MMPI) Profiles in Women Seeking Help for Premenstrual Syndrome*

Normal	36%
Neurotic	31%
Unclassified	17%
Characterological	11%
Psychotic	5%

*From Herzberg B, Coppen A: Changes in psychological symptoms in women taking oral contraceptives. *Brit J Psychiat* 1970; 116:161–164.

with the patient and spouse together to assess marital satisfaction and support systems. Problem areas in a marital relationship are often present throughout the month, but may tend to become more disruptive premenstrually.

Causes and Treatments of PMS

We will discuss the causes and treatments of PMS together, since etiologic hypotheses have logically led to attempts at treatment.

Studies of PMS treatment are often difficult to interpret. Most studies do not provide sufficient data on psychiatric assessment and many other aspects of subject selection to allow comparison among studies. In the absence of biochemical or physical markers of PMS, subjective changes in symptoms must be measured, many of which are internally perceived and not externally or objectively observable. In a manner similar to other studies dependent on a subjective evaluation of efficacy, most studies of drugs in the treatment of PMS have revealed a 25 percent to 50 percent nonspecific response to treatment.

To complicate matters further, clinical experience indicates that combinations of treatments often work better than any single treatment. Attribution of benefit to any single intervention or medication is therefore often difficult. Nevertheless, we will review the treatments most often used and discuss their value.

Nutrition

Many women complain of distinct food cravings premenstrually, usually for sweet or salty foods. There is some evidence that glucose tolerance increases premenstrually. Diabetics often have trouble regulating their insulin requirements during this time. There is some thought that reactive hypoglycemia may be more common in people with premenstrual syndrome.

Although nutrition in PMS remains incompletely investigated, there is some evidence[13] that people with premenstrual syndrome symptoms in fact eat a less well balanced diet than those without symptoms. For these reasons we and others have found it useful to suggest certain dietary modifications to treat PMS.

We suggest that a person should eat a balanced diet with meals spaced throughout the day. The diet should have a normal amount of protein, fat, and carbohydrates with emphasis being placed on complex carbohydrates rather than foods with high sugar content and refined carbohydrates. In addition, we recommend avoiding caffeine-containing foods and beverages and other central nervous system stimulants.

Although many women report feelings of bloatedness premenstrually, careful study has failed to document significant weight gain premenstrually in most women.[14] There may, however, be a shift of fluid into soft tissues, accounting for a sense of swelling in the extremities.[15] For this reason, we discourage the use of diuretics but do find it useful for a person to be careful about avoiding excess sodium intake especially during the premenstrual time.

Considerable attention has been paid to the role of micronutrients in PMS. We generally recommend a single generic multivitamin/multimineral supplement. There is no valid proof that special supplements containing large amounts of such elements as zinc and magnesium have any additional benefit in treating premenstrual symptoms.

Vitamin supplements are frequently recommended for PMS. Vitamin B_6, or pyridoxine, is known to be an important cofactor in many biosynthetic pathways in the body, including those involving neurotransmitters. In addition, controlled studies show[16] that vitamin B_6 will relieve depression symptoms in women taking birth control pills. For these reasons vitamin B_6 has been used to treat PMS. There are several studies showing some efficacy.[17,18]

Most studies have used vitamin B_6 at 100mg per day and for this reason we adhere to this dose level. Neurotoxicity has been observed in men and women using more than 2,000mg daily[19] and in one woman taking 500mg daily. Although there is no evidence suggesting toxicity at lower doses, we have maintained the 100mg per day limit out of caution.

Vitamin E has been described as helpful for the treatment of premenstrual mastalgia as well for relief of pain from fibrocystic changes in general. Although there is again some confusion in this area, several controlled studies support its use of 400 units per day.

Exercise

Much research has been done recently about the effects of exercise on brain function and mood in general. It seems effective in treating some forms of depression, and there are frequent subjective clinical reports that it helps to relieve the symptoms of premenstrual syndrome as well. Etiologic speculations center upon increased endorphin production during exercise, which may be important in both the regulation of mood and the perception of pain. For these reasons, as well as for the "break" from general life stresses that exercise often provides, we suggest regular daily exercise for women experiencing PMS.

Exercise may also help combat the effects of sleep disturance that sometimes appear premenstrually. Altered sleep patterns that accompany PMS and depression may be the cause of the general arthralgias commonly reported.

Life-style

Of the problems reported by our patients, the most common is the feeling of "not being able to cope with ordinary demands." One of the most helpful things about charting one's own symptoms is that it becomes possible to predict the most difficult days. With this in mind, it may be possible to schedule some optional activities that are stressful for the times when the fewest symptoms are present.

One of the easiest suggestions to make, but perhaps one of the hardest to follow, is for a person to allow a bit of time for herself, even on the most stressful days. Whether in the form of simply being alone, taking the time for a leisurely bath, a brief walk, or whatever activity is seen as relaxing, such a "break" can give a welcome respite from this feeling of being unable to cope. Legitimizing such activity as a prescription may help solicit family support.

Many couples find that they have disagreements that repeatedly emerge during premenstrual times. Often the discussion becomes heated to the point that productive problem solving cannot take place. In such situations, often the best thing a couple can do is to simply agree to stop the discussion when it has become unproductive, with the agreement to return to the issue when moods are calmer, perhaps in the first half of the next cycle. It is important, however, that the issues raised premenstrually not be dropped entirely or dismissed as being unimportant or coming "out of thin air." Rather, more useful problem solving can be undertaken when both people can approach the issue more calmly.

Some couples have found the premenstrual time to be useful to them in a very positive way. They find that the increased feelings of sensitivity at this time can make them aware of disagreements or issues between them that they might not have otherwise been able to detect. They can then use this insight productively, a process that may also require professional guidance.

Hormonal Treatments

Much has been said and written about the role of hormones in causing premenstrual symptoms. There is a current trend away from regarding PMS as due to deficiency or excess of a single steroid hormone, to implicating more complex central neuroregulatory disturbances.

Nevertheless, hormonal treatments have been used effectively as *medications* (not as replacement for a "deficiency"), and are often employed when the measures described so far are not sufficiently helpful. The two general types of hormone treatments that are used are those that 1) eliminate or suppress a women's endogenous hormone cycles, and 2) those that supplement a woman's endogenous hormones.

In the first group, those treatments that suppress or eliminate ovarian cyclicity are oral contraceptives, continuous medroxyprogesterone, danocrine, hysterectomy and bilateral oophorectomy, estrogen implants with the cyclic use of progesterone or various progestins, and finally recent experimental work with a gonadotropin releasing hormone (GnRH) agonist. We will discuss each of these individually.

Oral contraceptives will reduce premenstrual syndrome symptoms in general.[20] However, some women with more severe premenstrual depression will be at high risk for worsened premenstrual depression on the pill. About half of women who notice worsening depression on the pill will have that depression relieved by taking about 50mg of vitamin B_6 daily.[16] However, it has been suggested that the birth control pill will always aggravate PMS symptoms.[21] Empiric evidence is lacking for the argument that the pill makes a woman more likely to have worse PMS symptoms after discontinuing it. In our own clinic, we suggest the birth control pill for those who have experienced no negative side effects from them in the past and for whom no other contraceptive method is as appropriate.

Medroxyprogesterone acetate (Provera^R), an oral progestin, has been used by some clinicians to treat PMS, but apparently with mixed success. Although some studies show no effect, numerous clinicians have reported that some people do quite well on it while others find their depression aggravated. Our experience agrees with this and we do recommend it only occasionally. We discourage the use of the injectable form of medroxyprogesterone acetate due to its prolonged bioavailability.

Removal of the ovaries certainly brings about some relief of PMS symptoms in some physicians' experience. However, there are no published reports documenting this, and most clinicians feel that this is rather drastic treatment for a disorder that can often be quite effectively treated medically. Hormonal replacement with cyclic estrogen and progestins can be associated with a return of some of the symptoms of PMS, although usually to a less severe degree.[22]

In England, several physicians have used implanted pellets containing estradiol and cyclic oral progestins for 10 to 14 days out of each cycle. However, they have also observed the return of PMS symptoms where progestins are added. This approach has not been approved for use in this country.

Finally, recent work with gonadotropin releasing hormone (GnRH) agonist[23] has demonstrated once more that if you shut down the function of the ovaries, premenstrual symptoms will disappear. However, the increased risk of osteoporosis with this "medical oophorectomy" makes it inappropriate for general clinical use.

Danocrine has been employed with some anecdotal success, but is usually accompanied by significant untoward side effects. The safety of long-term use is unknown.

In general, although the treatments listed above are somewhat effective, they work by eliminating the menstrual cycle rather than adjusting or treating it in order to control symptoms. Our philosophy is that this is perhaps more meddlesome than hormone supplementation therapy as described below.

Dr. Katherina Dalton of England has been the most vocal proponent of progesterone supplementation therapy for treatment of PMS.[21] There is now a growing experience in this country with this medication including the work done in our clinic. Although controlled studies[24,25] have not shown progesterone to be beneficial, many clinics using it find that the apparent effectiveness of the medication in some women lasts much longer than the 2 to 3 months of response one would expect from a placebo. While awaiting further scientific studies to demonstrate its role, many clinics are continuing to use it, usually in the form of suppositories or a rectally administered suspension.

Progesterone supplementation therapy is usually confined to the second half of the menstrual cycle, starting at the beginning of symptoms, or at or around the time of ovulation and continuing until approximately day 27 or 28 of the cycle.

We have obtained encouraging results with 200mg to 400mg per day in two divided doses, using polyethylene glycol (PEG) base suppositories. Our limited experience in seeing patients using higher doses indicates that they did not reach significantly high blood levels with very large doses (1200 to 2400mg/day). Research is currently being conducted to investigate nasal delivery of progesterone.

When using these various hormonal measures to treat PMS symptoms, it is important to keep in mind that they are medications to treat symptoms and not the replacement for a known hormone deficiency. In this light, one might reach a point when other measures become more effective and hormone treatment is no longer required.

Other Medications

Aside from the hormonal and nutritional medications already mentioned, numerous other drugs have been used. We mentioned briefly that diuretics are widely used although they are of no proven benefit. The only diuretic that has any evidence supporting its effectiveness in PMS is spironolactone.[26] Used in amounts between 50mg and 100mg daily, some women find it effective. We generally have used this only when true weight gain has been documented by daily records, in order to avoid the possible hazzards of excess diuretic use. Improvement with spironolactone has been modest at best, perhaps because of the referral basis for our clinic.

Psychoactive drugs, including anxiolytics and antidepressants have also been used in PMS. Although studies of these drugs in PMS are few and not encouraging, we have found them useful in several ways. First, anxiolytics can be used intermittently if the most severe symptoms are of short duration. Side effects of somnolence and the potential for habituation with anxiolytics may make progesterone a more desirable option for women with symptoms lasting a week or more.

Antidepressants are of value primarily when prospective daily records indicate some evidence of month-long depression that worsens premenstrually. On occasion antidepressants are used in combination with progesterone. We will employ this combination only with psychiatric consultation and continued supervision.

Counseling

Many women experiencing premenstrual changes find that over months and years of having symptoms, their lives and relationships have been gradually eroded or damaged. The vicious interactive cycle of premenstrual symptoms and relationship stresses may often yield best to a combination of life change, diet, pharmacotherapy, and individual, family, or couples' therapy.

Premenstrual symptoms can also occur along with other disorders such as anxiety disorders, panic disorders, continuous depression, and manic-depressive illness. It is sometimes useful to combine both medical and psychological treatments of these problems with some of the treatments described above.

Support Groups

Women suffering from PMS in many cities throughout the country have gathered together to form support groups. These groups meet regularly to share their experiences in attempting to cope with PMS symptoms, and to share hints on dietary adjustments, exercise programs, problem solving techniques in their relationships, and finding appropriate sources of medical care. Such groups can be a valuable source of emotional and practical help in dealing with symptoms associated with PMS. They can also assist a woman in deciding when her symptoms are serious enough to require more comprehensive evaluation and treatment.

Several national groups maintain a roster of local support groups and sources of medical care for PMS. These include the National PMS Society, 3514 University Drive, Durham, NC 27707 and PMS Action, P. O. Box 19669, Irvine, CA 92713.

Medical Care for PMS

The essentials of evaluation, in our view, are 1) prospective daily ratings of symptoms, ideally by the person affected by PMS and by her partner or someone who is close to her, 2) review of diet and life-style, and 3) some assessment of personality, relationships, and general stresses and strains in life. When symptoms are not very severe, and/or when a physician knows his patient well, this can be effectively carried out in the primary care physician's office. When symptoms are more intense, or when more comprehensive evaluation seems appropriate, referral to a center with an established evaluation seems appropriate, referral to a center with an established evaluation program may be helpful, with a plan to return to the primary care physician for follow-up care at an appropriate time.

Summary

There is growing recognition that premenstrual changes may be triggered by definite (although poorly understood) chemical changes. At the same time, most clinicians dealing with premenstrual syndrome, and many women affected by it, also recognize that there are many ingredients in the mix, many factors that affect how a woman feels premenstrually. In the absence of a better understanding of etiology, we are limited to careful diagnosis followed by empiric treatment.

Hormonal and other drug treatments seem helpful and are most effective when used together with the diet and life-style changes mentioned. If life stresses can be reduced and unsolved problems worked out, it is sometimes possible to discontinue these medications and maintain symptom relief with the nonpharmacologic means. Counseling or therapy is useful for many. The growing research effort in PMS promises future improvements in this very important area of woman's health care.

References

1. Rubinow DR, Roy-Byrne P: Premenstrual syndrome: Overview from a methodologic perspective. Am J Psychiatry 1984; 141:163–171.
2. Clare AW: Psychologic profiles of women complaining of premenstrual symptoms. Curr Med Res Opin 1977; 4(Suppl 4):23–28.
3. Reid RL, Yen SSC: Premenstrual syndrome. Am J Obstet Gynecol 1985; 65:398–402.
4. Ruble DN: Premenstrual symptoms: A reinterpretation. Science 1977; 197:291–292.
5. Irwin J, Morge E, Riddick D: Dysmenorrhea induced by autologous infusion. Obstet Gynecol 1981; 58:286–290.
6. Halbreich U, Endicott J, Schacht S, Nee J: The diversity of premenstrual changes as reflected in the Premenstrual Assessment Form. Acta Psychiat Scand 1982; 65:46–65.

7. Herzberg B, Coppen A: Changes in psychological symptoms in women taking oral contraceptives. *Brit J Psychiat* 1970; 116:161–164.
8. Green R, Dalton K: The premenstrual syndrome. *Br Med J* 1953; 1:1007.
9. Steege JF, Stout AL, Rupp SL: Relationships among premenstrual symptoms and menstrual cycle characteristics. *Obstet Gynecol* 1985; 65:398–402.
10. Stout AL, Steege JF: Psychological assessment of women seeking treatment for premenstrual syndrome. *J Psychosom Res*, in press.
11. Hammond DC, Keye WR: Premenstrual syndrome (letter). *N Engl J Med* 1985; 312:920.
12. Beck AT: *Depression: Clinical, Experimental and Theoretical Aspects.* New York, Holber, 1967.
13. Abraham GE: Premenstrual tension. *Current Problems in Obstetrics and Gynecology* 1981; 3:1–39.
14. Faratian B, Gaspar A, O'Brien PMS et al: Premenstrual syndrome: Weight, abdominal swelling, and perceived body image. *Am J Obstet Gynecol* 1984; 150:200–204.
15. Wong WH, Freedman RI, Levan NE et al: Changes in capillary filtration coefficient of cutaneous vessels in women with premenstrual tension. *Am J Obstet Gynecol* 1972; 114:950–953.
16. Adams PW, Rose DP, Folkard J et al: Effect of pyridoxine hydrocholoride (vitamin B_6) upon depression associated with oral contraception. *Lancet* 1973; 1:897–904.
17. Derr GE: The management of premenstrual syndrome. *Curr Med Res Opin* 1977; 4(Suppl 4):29–34.
18. Abraham GE, Hargrove JT: Effect of vitamin B-6 on premenstrual symptomatology in women with premenstrual tension syndrome: A double-blind crossover study. *Infertility* 1980; 3:155–165.
19. Schaumburg H, Kaplan J, Windeband A et al: Sensory neuropathy from pyridoxine abuse. *N Engl J Med* 1983; 309:445–448.
20. Kutner SJ, Brown WL: Types of oral contraceptives, depression, and premenstrual symptoms. *J New Ment Dis* 1972; 155:153–162.
21. Dalton K: Charles C Thomas, Springfield IL, *The Premenstrual Syndrome.* 1964.

22. Hammarback S, Bachstrom T, Holst J et al: Cylical mood changes as in the premenstrual syndrome during sequential estrogen-progestogen postmenopausal replacement therapy. *Acta Obstet Gynecol Scand*, in press.
23. Muse KN, Futterman LA et al: The premenstrual syndrome: Effects of "medical oophorectomy." *N Engl J Med* 1984; 311:1345–1349.
24. Sampson GA: Premenstrual syndrome: A double-bind controlled trial of progesterone and placebo. *Br J Psychiatry* 1979; 135:209–215.
25. Smith SL: Mood and the menstrual cycle. In Sachar EJ (Ed), *Topics in Psychoendocrinology*. New York, Raven Press, 1975, pp. 19–58.
26. O'Brien PMS, Craven D, Selby C et al: Treatment of premenstrual syndrome by spironolactone. *Br J Obstet Gynecol* 1979; 86:142–147.

Chapter 4

FIBROMYALGIA

A Disorder for All Physicians

John R. Rice, M.D.

An understanding of the concept of fibromyalgia is of practical importance to virtually all clinicians who deal with pain-related complaints. The distinction between symptoms of psychological and psychophysiological origin is blurred in the minds of some physicians and, as a result, there is a substantial group of patients in almost any practice who may run the risk of less than optimal diagnostic and therapeutic management. Fibromyalgia serves admirably as a subject of discussion in clarifying this issue since it occurs frequently in a variety of practice settings, causes significant problems in terms of human suffering and disability, and there is an expanding body of information in the medical literature allowing a reasonable understanding of pathophysiology and therapy. The following case history illustrates a "typical" patient with fibromyalgia and will be a familiar story to many readers.

CASE REPORT

A woman I saw in clinic came for evaluation of what she had been told was "arthritis." When asked what bothered her most she replied, "I hurt all over," and, on closer questioning, indicated that for several years she had been having increasingly severe pain and soreness over most of her body. Her neck and shoulders, arms, elbows, upper back, chest wall, hips, and legs had all become involved. These areas ached, were sore to touch or pressure, and she described swelling in several locations. The pains were especially troublesome at night and she awakened in the morning exhausted to the point that she felt as if she "hadn't slept at all." She was so tired during the day that she had begun to notice problems with her memory and ability to concentrate. Her husband and children had complained that she had become unreasonably irritable.

She had been to her doctor at home and had taken a number of "arthritis" medications without benefit. Each seemed to help "a little at first," but her symptoms had continued to worsen. Her doctor had done a number of tests and X rays but could find "nothing wrong." She had brought records from her previous evaluations and, indeed, the tests and X rays had shown no indication of osteoarthritis, rheumatoid arthritis, lupus, or other specific disease process to explain her symptoms. She complained that she (and her doctor) was beginning to "feel like it's all in my head!"

On examination, her joints were not warm or swollen and moved easily through a full range of motion. She did, however, indicate significant tenderness on pressure over a number of areas in nearby soft tissues. On questioning, she indicated that her pains were not necessarily localized to the joints themselves but rather seemed to be "in the muscles or the bones," or "in the flesh," at times.

She agreed to having a few further laboratory studies done to make certain that we would not overlook any problems that might cause "all-over" discomfort. The test results were all normal. When she returned to clinic to review the results of her evaluation I told her that my diagnosis was "fibromyalgia," a very common and highly treatable cause of chronic pain that would not cause "crippling." With appropriate therapy she resolved the bulk of her symptoms within a few days. On a follow-up clinic visit 4 weeks later she reported complete relief of pain, stating that she "hadn't felt this good in years!"

Terminology

The story above brings to light one of the major problems in discussing fibromyalgia—terminology. There are few entities in clinical medicine for which there is a wider, and perhaps less appropriate, range of terms. I told the patient that she had fibromyalgia; another physician might have called it "rheumatic pain modulation disorder"; yet another might have diagnosed "chronic pain syndrome." A few would have unfortunately concluded that the woman was "crazy" or, worse yet, would have said that there was "nothing wrong" at all. A partial listing of some of the more common terms used synonymously with "fibromyalgia" is shown in Table 4-1.

As evidence has mounted to indicate that fibromyalgia is not a primary disorder of fibrous tissue or muscle, the obviously inappropriate nature of the term has produced several attempts at reform as listed above. Use of "fibromyalgia" and "fibrositis" remains in vogue, however, and is likely to persist in light of historical perspectives and because they are somewhat descriptive from a symptomatic standpoint.

Historical Perspectives

To understand and perhaps accept the problems of terminology encountered in a discussion of fibromyalgia it is nec-

Table 4-1. Fibromyalgia— Alternative Terminology

1. Fibrositis (syndrome)
2. Primary/secondary fibrositis
3. Myofascial pain syndrome
4. Rheumatic pain modulation disorder
5. Fibromyositis
6. Myofibrositis
7. Interstitial myofibrositis
8. Myofascitis
9. Chronic pain syndrome

essary to review the subject from an historical perspective. The term "fibrositis" was used initially by Gowers in 1904[1]. In a discourse on lumbago, he proposed that an exudative disorder of paralumbar fibrous tissues could explain the symptoms of this disorder, and suggested the term "fibrositis" to encompass this entirely hypothetical process. In the same year, Stockman[2] reported abnormal histological findings on biopsy of tender, nodular areas of soft tissue in patients with otherwise unexplained chronic rheumatic pains. Other reports followed in which patients with aches and pains were said to have tender areas of soft tissue nodularity varying in size and location depending on the patient population described. The term "fibrositis" fell into common diagnostic usage in these poorly defined groups of patients.

Attempts by subsequent investigators to reproduce Stockman's findings have failed. Biopsy of soft tissues in tender areas of patients with similar clinical pictures have shown, at best, nonspecific and minor alterations in histology. Areas of asymptomatic soft tissue nodularity are commonly found on close examination of "normal" subjects and areas of soft-tissue tenderness in patients with chronic pain syndromes are often unrelated to any palpable abnormalities in surrounding tissue[3]. The term "trigger point" came into usage briefly in describing areas of tenderness in these patients but has given way to "tender point" in the recent literature. In spite of disenchantment with the "nodules" described by Stockman, the medical community continues to be confronted with substantial numbers of patients with remarkably consistent complaints of significant and seemingly unexplained pain in association with predictable areas of soft-tissue tenderness. Regardless of uncertainties as to pathophysiology, the similarity of complaints and findings from patient to patient warrants designation as a syndrome. The terms "fibromyalgia" and "fibrositis" have served in this function in spite of attempts, as outlined above, to improve on terminology.

DIAGNOSTIC CRITERIA

There is no diagnostic "test" for fibromyalgia. The symptoms and findings are, however, highly characteristic and allow prompt clinical recognition. Criteria for a diagnosis of "primary fibromyalgia" (PF), formulated by the controlled study of Yunus et al.[4] are outlined in Table 4-2.

The "tender points" in the criteria of Yunus et al. refer to the localized areas of soft-tissue tenderness found on a standardized examination of patients with fibromyalgia. Characteristic anatomical regions where tender points are most commonly located are shown in Figure 4-1. A female figure is used since roughly 80 percent of patients with fibromyalgia are women.

Given the lack of correlation with objective abnormality in

Table 4-2. Primary Fibromyalgia—Suggested Criteria*

1. Obligatory
    a. generalized aches and pains (or prominent stiffness)
        1) minimum of 3 anatomical sites
        2) minimum of 3 months' duration
    b. absence of coexistent "secondary" disorders
        1) traumatic injury
        2) structural rheumatic disease (osteoarthritis, etc.)
        3) infectious arthritis
        4) endocrine-related arthropathy
        5) abnormal laboratory tests (positive ANA, etc.)
2. Major—5 or more typical and consistent "tender points"
3. Minor
    a. alteration in symptoms with activity
    b. alteration in symptoms with weather
    c. alteration in symptoms with anxiety/stress
    d. inadequate sleep
    e. generalized fatigue
    f. anxiety
    g. headache
    h. irritable bowel syndrome
    i. subjective "swelling" in symptomatic areas
    j. nonsegmental, nonradicular "numbness"

Diagnosis—obligatory criteria + 1 major or minor criteria

*From Yunus M, Masi AT, Calabro JJ et al: Primary fibromyalgia (fibrositis): Clinical study of 50 patients with matched normal controls. *Semin Arthritis Rheum* 1981; 11:151–171.

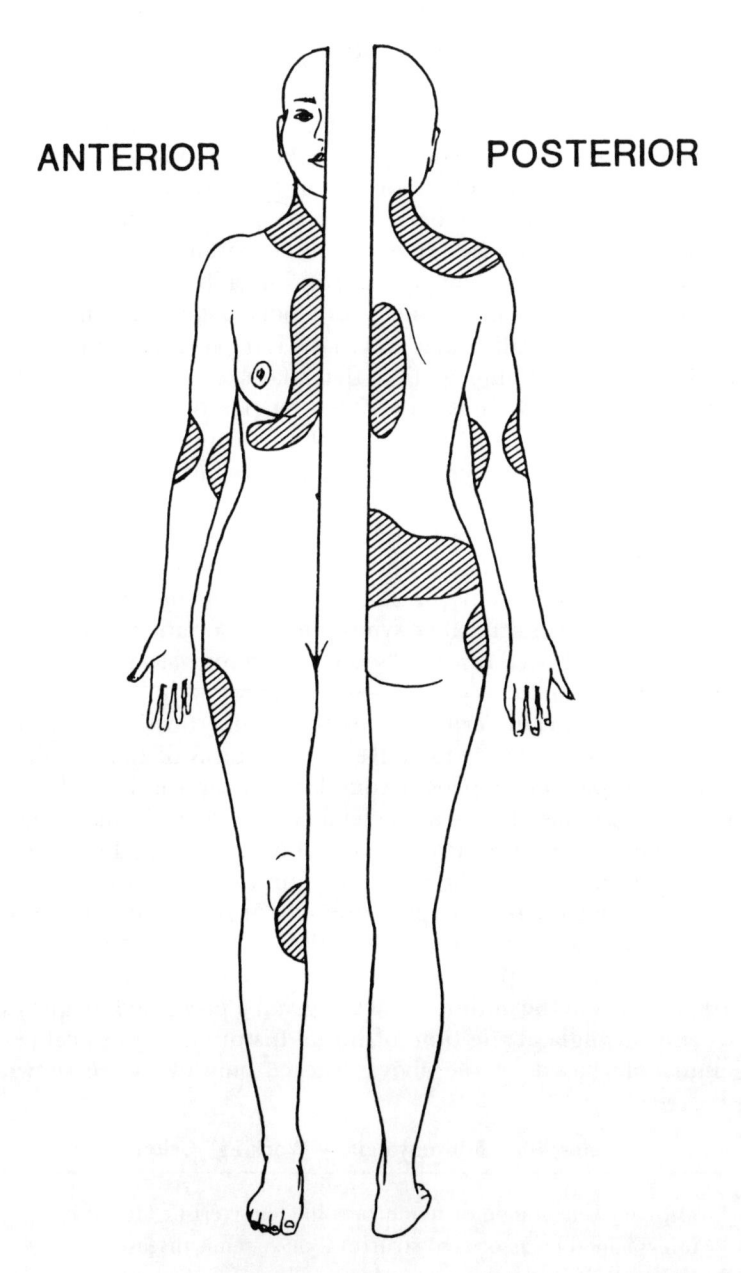

Figure 4-1. Tender points—common anatomical locations in fibromyalgia.

the area of tenderness, this "finding" represents subjective information dependent somewhat on the skills of the examiner and the completeness of examination. In a given patient, however, tender points have been shown to be highly consistent on serial evaluation by the same examiner. Yunus et al., in their comparison of 50 patients with fibromyalgia to normal controls, demonstrated that small numbers of tender points are commonly found in normal individuals and that it is the increased numbers of these areas in a single patient that characterizes fibromyalgia. Their study found a mean of 12 tender points in patients with PF (range 4-38) versus a mean of 1.1 in controls (range 0-4). They suggested a minimum of 5 tender points as a diagnostic criterion.

Although important for careful selection of a patient population in clinical studies, criteria like those above are somewhat unwieldly in day-to-day practice and exclude the common occurrence of fibromyalgialike symptoms in association with structural musculoskeletal disease ("secondary fibromyalgia"). Broader and more streamlined guidelines are suggested in Table 4-3.

These "working criteria" reflect the diagnostic algorithm used in clinical practice to arrive at a diagnosis of fibromyalgia in a given patient: A patient complains of significant and persistent symptoms of musculoskeletal pain in multiple anatomical area; there are no objective anatomical or physiological disorders found on subsequent physical, laboratory, and radiographic examination adequate to explain the extent or degree of symptomatology; and the patient describes chronic fatigue and/or nonrestorative sleep in association with the pain. In a review of 100 patients in the author's practice given a presumed diagnosis of fibromyalgia at the time of initial history and physical examination, based on the above criteria, only two were shown

Table 4-3. Fibromyalgia—"Working" Criteria

1. Musculoskeletal pain or tenderness in characteristic locations unexplained by associated structural or systemic disease.
2. Duration of symptoms > 3 months.
3. Associated sleep disturbance or chronic fatigue.

eventually to have an alternative diagnosis to explain their symptoms and this became apparent immediately on return of initial laboratory studies. One of the patients had early rheumatoid arthritis and the other, early symptoms of giant-cell arteritis. None of the other 98 patients over a minimum of 2 years' follow-up had a change in diagnosis.

Associated Symptomatology

Symptoms other than musculoskeletal pain commonly accompany the syndrome of fibromyalgia and have been well described and tabulated by Yunus et al.[4] and other authors. Fatigue and a disturbance in sleep are described by virtually all patients. Problems with memory and concentration are frequent, along with varying degrees of depression and irritability. Diffuse hyperreflexia is a common finding on physical examination. Patients often describe a history of "growing pains" in childhood, and may have a long history of severe headaches and/or "irritable bowel syndrome." A history of urinary urgency or frequency may be obtained. Subjective complaints of "swelling" in affected parts, not apparent to the examining physician, may occur and patients often describe acroparesthesia or dysesthesia in the face of a normal neurological examination.

Pathophysiology

The first significant investigations into the pathophysiology of fibromyalgia began with the studies of Moldofsky et al. in 1975[5] and 1976[6]. They monitored sleep patterns by EEG in patients with fibromyalgia and demonstrated a relative absence of an alphalike intrusion in Stages 3 and 4 of non-REM sleep. They then produced symptoms similar to fibromyalgia in normal subjects by selective deprivation of Stage 3 and 4 sleep; similar deprivation of REM sleep in normal subjects roduced no untoward effects. They postulated a possible role of disturbed central nervous system (CNS) function in the pathophysiology of fibromyalgia. Extrapolating from a review of reports by other authors of pain syndromes both in animal experiments and in man produced by inhibition of CNS serotonin, they postulated a disturbance of serotonin pathways in the production of pain in fibromyalgia.

In further studies they found reduced plasma tryptophan levels in patients with fibromyalgia[7]. They gave oral 1-tryptophan to patients with fibromyalgia with subsequent reduced sleep latency and improved Stage 2 non-REM sleep but with no increase in Stage 3 and 4 sleep and no improvement in symptoms; chlorpromazine was shown to increase Stages 3 and 4 non-REM sleep in similar subjects with associated improvement in mood and pain[8]. Serotonergic tricylics have come into increasingly widespread usage by the medical community in the management of various pain syndromes and, in the author's practice, have proven to be of sometimes dramatic benefit in 50 percent or more of patients with fibromyalgia.

The role of psychological factors in fibrositis is a subject of major controversy. Multiple studies have shown a significant component of depression in patients with fibrositis[9,10]. Of major importance, however, is the consistent absence of affective manifestations of depression in approximately one-third of these patients[11]. Smythe further points out the problems inherent in applying the commonly used affective indices to patients with pain-producing disorders[12]. The distinction between the highly consistent complaints and findings of fibromyalgia, and the bizarre, highly variable aspects of "conversion hysteria" or "psychogenic rheumatism" is evident to the most casual examiner.

Several authors have commented on the personality profile characteristic of fibromyalgia: the extra hard-working individual, with somewhat rigid concepts of proper social and ethical behavior, who "never missed a day of work" and who never learned to say "no" to demands of others. Smythe summarized this nicely by pointing out that these patients "are not abnormal, only characteristic"[13]. Many authors have noted an apparent role of "stress" in the symptomatology of fibrositis; in the author's practice it has seemed that "stress" in these patients is most commonly of intrinsic origin, a product primarily of personality rather than of environmental problems per se. Further clarification of these issues will await a more cooperative approach involving both rheumatologists and psychiatrists; but it seems reasonable to conclude that symptoms experienced by these patients are real and that personality structure and intrinsic behavior may play at least as important a role as "depression" in pathophysiology.

If one is willing to translate "stress" or "depression" into alterations of CNS function, based on physical demand at the tissue or neurochemical level, then a hypothetical construct of a possible (and undoubtedly partial) explanation of the pain and other features of fibromyalgia may be outlined as in Figure 4-2.

In this simplistic hypothesis, personality traits, extrinsic environmental pressures, chronic illness, etc., place a demand ("stress") on the CNS for excessive physiological function from the standpoint of both duration and intensity of function. Induced neuropharmacological changes, involving in part the serotonergic pathways, thus produced may cause impairment in function of portions of the CNS and result clinically in chronic fatigue, alterations in mood and cortical functions, disordered sleep and alterations of intrinsic pain modulation—i.e. "fibromyalgia." Anatomical features of peripheral and central pain

FIBROSITIS -- hypothesis

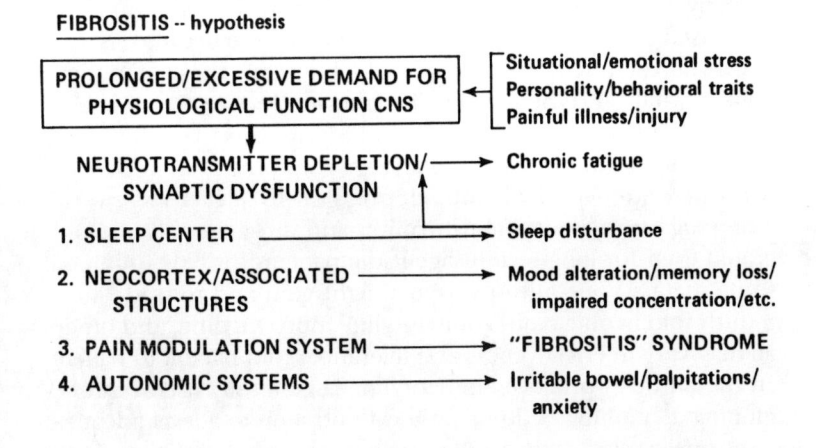

```
PROLONGED/EXCESSIVE DEMAND FOR  ←   Situational/emotional stress
  PHYSIOLOGICAL FUNCTION CNS         Personality/behavioral traits
              │                      Painful illness/injury
              ↓
  NEUROTRANSMITTER DEPLETION/  ──→  Chronic fatigue
     SYNAPTIC DYSFUNCTION
                          ↑
  1. SLEEP CENTER ────────┴──────→  Sleep disturbance

  2. NEOCORTEX/ASSOCIATED  ──────→  Mood alteration/memory loss/
        STRUCTURES                   impaired concentration/etc.

  3. PAIN MODULATION SYSTEM ─────→  "FIBROSITIS" SYNDROME

  4. AUTONOMIC SYSTEMS ──────────→  Irritable bowel/palpitations/
                                     anxiety
```

Figure 4-2. Fibromyalgia—hypothetical pathophysiology.

pathways, including the normally inhibitory functions of the endogenous pain modulation system, were reviewed in 1984[14] and are not inconsistent with the above hypothesis.

Therapy

The most straightforward initial approach to the treatment of fibromyalgia is pharmacological. In spite of the evident role of affective and personality factors in this disorder, the realities of clinical practice preclude the wholesale referral of these patients to either psychiatrists or to "stress and pain management centers." A reassuring and nonjudgmental approach by the primary physician, a reasonable amount of time invested in patient education, and a relatively simple therapeutic program will suffice to relieve the symptoms of most patients. The knowledge that their doctor "knows what is wrong" and that they "are not crazy" has a remarkably therapeutic effect on the patient who has had an unsatisfactory experience sometimes with several previous physicians.

An initial trial of aspirin or prescribed nonsteroidal, antiinflammatory agents (NSAID), coupled with simple physical therapy, may be beneficial in some patients with mild symptoms. Increased physical activity, structured or nonstructured, is very helpful if tolerated. Most frequently, however, these modalities help "at first" and then rapidly become ineffective. A single bedtime dose of one of the tricyclic antidepressants (TCAs) may be highly successful in rapidly relieving symptoms even in patients without evidence of obvious depression by affective criteria. These agents are not habit-forming and are generally well tolerated even for long-term usage if the patient is willing to impose some dietary control to prevent weight gain and to trade a dry mouth for chronic pain. Amitriptyline, nortriptyline, and others all may vary in effectiveness and tolerance from patient to patient. In the author's practice amitriptyline is generally used first, beginning at a 50 mg bedtime dose with titration to a level adequate to normalize sleep and produce maximal pain relief. Other TCAs may be substituted as indicated. Approximately 50 percent of patients will respond completely and another 25 percent partially to TCAs. A few will be able to discontinue therapy after a few weeks or months with no recurrence of symptoms; others will require intermittent or long-term maintenance therapy. Any of these possibilities are preferable to chronic uncontrolled pain. As with any class of drug, physicians need to be familiar with less common potential side effects and drug interactions before prescribing these agents.

The patient with fibromyalgia unresponsive to or intolerant of TCAs presents a difficult management problem. Injection of tender points with local anesthetics, with or without corticosteroids, has limited application. Protracted oral corticosteroid therapy has *no* role in the management of this disorder. EMG biofeedback has proven generally disappointing, frequent use of narcotic analgesics is undesirable, and the non-TCA antidepressants seem to function poorly in providing pain relief. A multidisciplinary pain management program may be the most satisfactory approach to these patients, offering at least some hope of helping them adjust to chronic pain.

REFERENCES

1. Gowers WR: Lumbago: Its lessons and analogues. *Br Med J* 1904;1:117–121.
2. Stockman R: The causes, pathology and treatment of chronic rheumatism. *Edinb Med J* 1904; 15:107–116, 223–235.
3. Smythe HA: Non-articular rheumatism and the fibrositis syndrome. In Hollander JI, McCarty DJ (Eds), *Arthritis and Allied Conditions,* 8th ed. Philadelphia, Lea and Febiger, 1972, pp.874–884.
4. Yunus M, Masi AT, Calabro JJ *et al:* Primary fibromyalgia (fibrositis): Clinical study of 50 patients with matched normal controls. *Semin Arthritis Rheum* 1981; 11:151–171.
5. Moldofsky H, Scarisbrick P, England R *et al:* Musculoskeletal symptoms and non-REM sleep disturbance in patients with "fibrositis syndrome" and healthy subjects. *Psychosom Med* 1975; 37:341–351.

6. Modofsky H, Scarisbrick P: Induction of neurasthenic musculoskeletal pain syndrome by selective sleep stage deprivation. *Psychosom Med* 1976; 38:35–44.
7. Moldofsky H, Warsh JJ: Plasma tryptophan and musculoskeletal pain in non-articular rheumatism. *Pain* 1978; 5:65–71.
8. Moldofsky H, Lue FA: The relationship of alpha and delta EEG frequencies to pain and mood in "fibrositis" patients treated with chlorpromazine and 1-tryptophan. *Electroencephal Clin Neurophysiol* 1980; 50:71–80.
9. Payne TC, Leavitt F, Garron DC *et al:* Fibrositis and psychologic disturbance. *Arthritis Rheum* 1982; 25:213–217.
10. Wolfe F, Cathey MA, Kleinheksel SM *et al:* Psychological status in primary fibrositis and fibrositis associated with RA. *J. Rheumatol* 1984; 11(4):500–506.
11. Ahles TA, Yunus MB, Riley SD *et al:* Psychological factors associated with primary fibromyalgia syndrome. *Arthritis Rheum* 1984; 27:1101–1106.
12. Smythe HA: Problems with the MMPI. *J Rheum Dis* 1984; 11:417–418.
13. Smythe HA: "Fibrositis" and other diffuse musculoskeletal syndromes. In Kelly WN, Harris ED, Ruddy SH *et al* (Eds), *Textbook of Rheumatology* 2nd ed. Philadelphia, WB Saunders, 1985, pp.481–489.
14. Fields HL: Neurophysiology of pain and pain modulation. *Am J Med* 1984; 77(3A):2–8.

Chapter 5

HEADACHES

E. Wayne Massey, M.D.

The clinician's most valuable diagnostic tool is usually a detailed history. For individuals with headache, this is especially true.

The history must be taken with genuine interest and concern, so the patient will feel encouraged to ventilate his problems. For many headache patients, there is a genuine fear of a brain tumor or other catastrophic illness, and the history may be distorted or certain points may be omitted. Specific concise points should be included in all headache histories.[1,2]

TYPES OF HEADACHE (TABLE 5-1)

It is essential to elicit from the patient how many types of headaches he can identify. Quite often, a patient with a long history of recurrent one-sided severe headaches will develop a daily constant headache. This may also be accompanied by a sleep disturbance, typical of depression.

In order to determine the type of headache, it is important to elicit the age of original onset. Vascular headaches usually

Table 5-1. Headache History

---

1. How many/type
2. Onset
3. Location
4. Timing
5. Frequency
6. Duration
7. Severity
8. Characteristics
9. Prodrome
10. Associated symptoms
11. Precipitating factor
12. Family history
13. Past medical history
14. Allergy history
15. Medication (past and present)

---

begin in childhood, adolescence, or the third and fourth decades. Those headaches that start in the fifth decade will usually have a psychogenic component, such as depression; however, organic disease must be ruled out.[3]

Determining the length of the illness is also important. A patient who notes a 10- to 40-year history of headache will usually not be suffering from an organic illness. A sudden onset of the headache with other neurological symptoms will alert the physician to a possible organic cause.

Precipitating factors should also be discussed. Headaches following a trauma will also require further evaluation. The female may note that the headaches started about the time of her menarche or may be related to pregnancy or menopause.

The site of the pain is essential in identifying the type of headache. Pain always localized on one side can be indicative of migraine or organic disease, unless the clinical features are typical of cluster headache, tic douloureux, or local changes in the eyes, sinuses, skull, or scalp. Generalized pain may indicate psychogenic components if there is no evidence of increased intracranial pressure. If the pain is localized to the eye alone, the physician should be suspicious of cluster headache or ocular disease. The "hatband" distribution of head pain is typical of headaches with psychogenic components. It is also important to note that migraine will switch sides.

In cluster headache, the patient will often complain of headache that will awaken him in the middle of the night and will continue for a few minutes to a few hours. The headache associated with hypertension is typically present on awakening and disappears as the day continues. In contrast, sinus headache starts gradually in the morning and will become worse as the day progresses.

Migraine occurs periodically, possibly once every 1 to 2 months. During pregnancy and vacations, migraine is often absent. However, many patients will complain of their headaches exclusively during vacations or on weekends. Cluster headaches are so named because of their occurrence in a series, lasting several weeks or months. These series most often appear in spring and fall. Occasionally, a patient with cluster headaches will complain of a chronic cluster headache. Muscle contraction headaches, seen by the headache clinician, are chronic in nature, and usually occur on a daily basis. Physical and neurological examinations on these patients are usually normal.

The pain of the headache due to an organic cause is usually persistent and progressively increases in intensity. Migraine headaches will continue from 6 hours to 3 days or longer. The pain will not be a constant ache, but rather intense pulsating or throbbing. Cluster headache will also be throbbing, is usually very severe, and is described as deep and boring. The duration of cluster headache is short, lasting from several minutes to 3 to 4 hours. A shocklike, stabbing pain is present in tic douloureux, is typically neuritic in character, and will last from only 1 to 15 minutes. Persistent, dull, and nagging pain is typical of headaches due to a psychogenic component, and the pain will increase occasionally.

Prodrome

Warning symptoms are typical of classical migraine, and will usually occur 40 to 60 minutes preheadache. The symptoms are most often visual in nature, such as zigzag flashing lights and colors, scotomata, or hemianopia. It is believed that these symptoms originate in the visual cortex portions of the occipital lobe. Other prodromata include strange odors, sensory phenomena such as paresthesias or hypothesias, vertigo, defects of mobility or coordination, oculomotor paralysis, or hemiparesis.

The visual disturbances may also occur with tumors or vascular disorders, such as an angioma. In some headache patients, as they grow older, the headache may diminish but the prodromata will continue to occur, without any headache following the visual symptoms.

Associated Symptoms

Migraine headaches are most often associated with nausea and vomiting. This is the reason migraine is described as a "sick headache." Other associated symptoms include: phonophobia, photophobia, blurred vision, dizziness, ringing in the ears, and focal neurologic changes. Patients with cluster headache will complain of facial flushing, lacrimation, and a nasal discharge associated with their headaches. These symptoms often occur on the same side as the headache. If a patient complains of double vision, convulsions, or tinnitus, an organic cause of the headache should be ruled out. Patients suffering from headaches with psychogenic components will have a long list of various somatic, emotional, and psychic symptoms.

Precipitating Factors

Many factors can precipitate migraine attacks, including fatigue, stress, menstruation, ovulation, lack of sleep, bright sunlight, too much sleep, alcohol, and change in weather and barometric pressure. Foods containing tyramine or sodium nitrite can be causative factors. In the "Chinese restaurant syndrome," monosodium glutamate can cause a vascularlike headache. It is common for migraine sufferers to create an environment impossible to handle. The stress resulting from this situation may trigger a headache. Drugs containing vasoactive materials may also induce a migraine.

Frequently, migraine first appears at the onset of menses. During pregnancy, migraine will disappear by the third month, but will reappear following the delivery of the child. Migraine often disappears with menopause. However, migraine may be prolonged if postmenopausal hormones are administered. In contrast, sometimes migraine that reappears at the time of menopause may be improved with the administration of estrogen therapy.

Headaches may be precipitated by the occupation of the sufferer. Munitions workers are exposed to nitrates, which cause vasodilation of the cerebral vessels and will resemble vascular headaches. Workers in poorly ventilated areas, such as mechanics, are exposed to carbon monoxide, which can trigger headaches. Headaches precipitated by exertion, such as straining or cough, are not necessarily associated with intracranial tumors, and are often benign. These benign exertional headaches can occur in conjunction with vascular headaches in some sufferers.

An inventory of emotional factors is essential in determining the psychological background of the headache sufferer. The patient should be carefully questioned regarding marital and family relationships, occupational, social, and environmental stresses, and any sexual difficulties. This discussion may allow the patient to ventilate any possible problems that would relate to his headaches. Since some patients will not communicate problems until they have become confident toward the interviewer, the questioning may need to be repeated on follow-up visits.

Patients with migraine and depressive headaches will often present a family history of headaches. Most experts concur that migraine is an hereditary disease. Prior history of head trauma may be present during the questioning of the patient's medical history. The patient may reveal a history of convulsions associated with headaches and neck stiffness which may be indicative of cerebral vascular malformation, such as an angioma, and so on. The previous medical history may also determine the therapy for the headache problem. For example, propranolol is contraindicated in patients with asthma. A history of a tumor may suggest the cancer has metastasized to the brain, triggering a headache. Obviously, history of any previous neurological surgery will alert the physician to rule out an organic cause of the headache.

Headache symptoms may be exacerbated or intensified in patients with seasonal allergies during the allergy season. However, no one has identified a specific antibody-antigen relationship to migraine.

Medications

If previous therapy with ergotamine therapy has helped the patient, the most likely diagnosis is migraine. If antidepressants have been effective, depression is indicated. It is essential, therefore, that a careful inventory of previous medications and their results should be included.

Obviously, the physician should be aware of the medications the patient is currently taking for headaches and other indications. For example, reserpine used in hypertension therapy may precipitate or increase the severity of migraine attacks. Oral contraceptive, postmenopausal hormones, and the nitrates used in coronary artery disease may induce migraine in susceptible patients.

MUSCLE CONTRACTION (TENSION) HEADACHES

Eighty percent of the headache patients seen by a general physician suffer from muscle contraction or tension headache. Which manifest in relationship to stress, depression, emotional conflicts, fatigue, or repressed hostility. These problems may not be evident to the sufferer.

Muscle contraction headaches can occur at any age but are more common in adulthood when the frustrations of life tend to dominate. The majority of patients are female and about 40 percent have a family history of headache, compared to 70 percent of migraine suffers. The usual onset of patients' headaches is between the ages of twenty and forty.

Muscle contraction headache may occur as a secondary phenomenon when there is head or face pain from other causes. Examples are headache associated with sustained muscle contraction due to faulty posture, cervical spondylosis, discogenic disease, bony anomalies of the occipital-cervical junction, cervical cord and posterior cranial fossa tumors, and disorders of the tempomandibular joint.

The tension headache is a steady, nonpulsatile ache. Additional descriptive terms include: "tightness" bitemporally or at the occiput; "bandlike" sensations about the head, which may become caplike in distribution; "viselike"; "weight"; "pressure"; "drawing"; and "soreness."

These head pains or other sensations occur frequently in the forehead and temples or in the back of the head and neck, as well as at other sites. They may be unilateral or bilateral, involving the temporal, occipital, parietal, or frontal regions, or any combination of these sites. Frequently, there is a soreness on combing or brushing the hair or when putting on a hat. (Table 5-2)

Table 5-2. Classification of Headache

1) Vascular headaches of migraine type. Recurrent attacks of headache, widely varied in intensity, frequency, and duration. The attacks are commonly unilateral in onset; are usually associated with anorexia and, sometimes with nausea and vomiting; in some are preceded by, or associated with, conspicuous sensory, motor, and mood disturbances; and are often familial.
   A. *"Classic" migraine.* Vascular headache with sharply defined, transient visual, and other sensory or motor prodromes or both.
   B. *"Common" migraine.* Vascular headache without striking prodromes and less often unilateral than A and C. Synonyms are "atypical migraine" or "sick headache."
   C. *"Cluster" headache.* Vascular headache, predominantly unilateral on the same side, usually associated with flushing, sweating, rhinorrhea, and increased lacrimation; brief in duration and usually occurring in closely packed groups separated by long remissions. Identical or closely allied are: ciliary or migrainous neuralgia, erythromelalgia of the head or histaminic cephalgia, and petrosal neuralgia.

Table 5-2. Classification of Headache *(Continued)*

- D. *"Hemiplegic" migraine and "ophthalmoplegic" migraine.* Vascular headache featured by sensory and motor phenomena which persist during and after the headache.
- E. *"Lower-half" headache.* Headache of possibly vascular mechanism, centered primarily in the lower face. In this group there may be some instances of "atypical facial" neuralgia, sphenopalatine ganglion neuralgia, and vidian neuralgia.

2) *Muscle contraction headache.* Usually an ache or sensations of tightness, pressure, or constriction, widely varied in intensity, frequency, and duration, sometimes long lasting, and commonly suboccipital. It is associated with sustained contraction of skeletal muscles in the absence of permanent structural change, usually as part of the individual's reaction during life stress.

3) *Combined headache: Vascular and muscle contraction.* Combinations of vascular headache of the migraine type and muscle contraction headache prominently coexisting in an attack.

4) *Headache of nasal vasomotor reaction.* Headaches and nasal discomfort (nasal obstruction, rhinorrhea, tightness or burning), recurrent and resulting from congestion and edema of nasal and paranasal mucous membranes, and not proven due to allergens, infectious agents, or local gross anatomic defects; predominantly anterior in location, and mild or moderate in intensity.

5) *Headache of delusional, conversion, or hypochondriacal states.* "Psychogenic" headaches of illnesses in which the prevailing clinical disorder is a delusional or a conversion reaction and a peripheral pain mechanism is nonexistent. Closely allied are the hypochondriacal reactions in which peripheral disturbances relevant to headache are minimal.

6) *Nonmigrainous vascular headaches.* These are associated with generally nonrecurrent dilatation of cranial arteries:
   - A. Systemic infections, usually with fever.
   - B. Miscellaneous disorders, including: hypoxic states; carbon monoxide poisoning; effects of nitrites, nitrates, and other chemical agents with vasodilator properties; caffeine withdrawal reaction; circulatory insufficiency in the brain (in certain circumstances); postconcussion reactions;

Table 5-2. Classification of Headache *(Continued)*

---

postconvulsive states; "hangover" reactions; foreign protein reactions; hypoglycemia; hypercapnia; acute pressor reactions (abrupt elevation of blood pressure, as with paraplegia or pheochromocytoma); and certain instances of essential arterial hypertension (e.g., those with early morning headache).

7) *Traction headache.* Headaches resulting from traction on intracranial vascular structures, by masses:
   A. Primary or metastatic tumors of meninges, vessels, or brain.
   B. Hematomas (epidural, subdural, or parenchymal).
   C. Abscesses (epidural, subdural, or parenchymal).
   D. Postlumbar puncture headache.
   E. Pseudotumor cerebri (or various causes of brain swelling).
8) *Headache due to overt cranial inflammation.* Headaches due to readily recognized inflammation of cranial structures, resulting from usually nonrecurrent inflammation, sterile or infectious.
9) Headache due to spread of effects of noxious stimulation of ocular structures (as by increased intraocular pressure excessive contraction of ocular muscles, trauma, new growth, or inflammation).
10) Headache due to spread of effects of noxious stimulation of aural structure (as by trauma, new growth, or inflammation).
11) Headache due to spread of effects of noxious stimulation of nasal and sinusal structures (as by trauma, new growth, inflammation, or allergens).
12) Headache due to spread of effects of noxious stimulation of dental structures (as by trauma, new growth, or inflammation).
13) Headache due to speread of pain from noxious stimulation of other structures of the cranium and neck (periosteum, joint, ligaments, muscles, or cervical roots).
14) *Cranial neuritides.* Caused by trauma, new growth, or inflammation.
15) *Cranial neuralgias.* Trigeminal (tic douloureux) and glossopharyngeal. The pains are lancinating ("jabbing"), usually in rapid succession for several minutes or longer, are limited to a portion or all of the domain of a cranial nerve (V or IX).

Although muscle contraction headache may be fleeting, with frequent changes in the site and intensity, this is the type of headache which, localized in one region, may be sustained with varying intensity for weeks, months, or years. The intensity of the headache may be diminished by assuming certain individually favored positions. The patient may limit the motion of the head, neck, and jaws because it decreases his discomfort.

Within the diffusely aching muscle tissues of the head, neck, and upper back, there may be found on palpation one or more tender areas, or nodules, which are sharply localized. Such pressure on tender areas causes radiation of the pain to adjacent portions of the head. Muscle contraction headache may also be aggravated by shivering from exposure to cold.

The physiological response that follows is a reflex dilatation of the external cranial vessels and a contraction of the skeletal muscles of the head, neck, or face, resulting in the characteristic pain of muscle contraction headache.

The amount of muscle tone at the head and scalp are determined by the degree of activity of a special group of anterior horn cells called the fusimotor or gamma efferent neurons. A small inhibitory nerve cell called the Renshaw cell acts on the alpha motor neurons supplying the extrafusal fibers. The cortical, afferent, and efferent pathways are also directly related to these symptoms, and it is the interreaction between these symptoms that maintains the state of muscle tone. The excessive muscle contraction producing the pain leads to anxiety and reinforces the excessive muscle contraction, thereby starting a vicious and self-sustaining circle.

Inquiring if the patient has chronic feelings of tension, nervousness, irritability, or difficulty relaxing is important. Since headache often accompanies depression, a careful inventory of depressive symptoms should be taken. The depressed patient may exhibit many physical symptoms such as headache, sleep disturbance, shortness of breath, constipation, weight loss, feelings of fatigue, decreased sexual drive, palpitations, and menstrual changes. Some patients will cry spontaneously as one talks to them. They will express feelings of guilt, hopelessness, unworthiness, and unreality, and may have some anxiety along with their depression. There may be a basic fear of insanity, physical disease or death, and these patients will ruminate over the past, present, and future. Psychic complaints may present, such as poor concentration, loss of interest, ambition, indecisiveness, poor memory, and suicidal thoughts. These patients view morning as the worst time of the day and may have a diurnal variation to their pain.

There are two types of muscle contraction headache: episodic and chronic. The episodic type is quite common, and many of these patients never seek the help of a physician since their headaches are relieved by various over-the-counter analgesics. A problem starts when the analgesics are taken on a daily basis or in excessive amounts. The characteristics of the episodic muscle contraction headaches are mild to moderate pain involving the temporal, frontal, vertex or occipital, and cervical regions separately or in any combination. The headaches are usually described as occurring bilaterally and may be triggered by such factors as fatigue, acute family crisis, and stressful work loads.

Chronic muscle contraction headache is constant and unremitting. It may be present for weeks, months, years, or decades. The pain may affect the same areas of the head as the acute type and is characteristically bilateral. Some patients describe a "tight band," like a tight skullcap, or hatband distribution to the headache.

If the headache occurs on an intermittent basis, the treatment of the muscle contraction headache includes common analgesics. Sometimes a thorough history and a neurological examination may be all the reassurance a patient requires. If there are psychological problems, an inventory should be made of their psychogenic determinants (Table 5-2).

The tricyclic antidepressants are probably the most useful of all therapeutic agents. If anxiety is a primary factor, the addition of a mild tranquilizer with the tricyclic antidepressant may be indicated. Propranolol is sometimes helpful and can be used in combination with the tricyclic compounds. It has been shown to have an anxiolytic effect, which may explain its beneficial response. If the patients present with a mixed headache syndrome—vascular headache with tension headache—propranolol may be especially beneficial in these cases.

Biofeedback can[4,5] be of great value in the patient with muscle contraction headaches who is not depressed. It is important to use biofeedback in intelligent patients and in patients who are not averse to participating in a method to train physiological functions. The purpose of biofeedback in the treatment of muscle contraction headache is to train the patients to use their thought process through electromyographic relaxation techniques in order to override the physiological disturbance that occurs with this disorder.

Vascular Headaches

Classical migraine, common migraine, cluster headaches, hemiplegic or ophthalmoplegic migraine and lower half headaches (Sluder's neuralgia) are common. They may also be classified as the premonitory migraine, the prodromal migraine, migraine equivalents, nonprodromal migraine, and complicated migraine. Some patients have premonitory complaints or symptoms. These individuals feel depressed or anxious for 24 hours or may have an increased appetite before a headache begins. They know within 24 hours when they are going to have a headache.

Prodromal migraine may be divided into classic or protracted prodromal migraine. Classic migraine has focal neurological symptoms or signs which disappear before the migraine begins. Often these focal findings, either scintillations, scotomata, unilateral numbness, or weakness aphasia does not go away prior to the headache, so is "protracted." These are more common than the classic type. Migraine equivalents occur in individuals with prodromal symptoms but no headache. These are difficult to diagnose except by exclusion. Transient migraine accompaniments occur in older individuals who have scotoma, or scintillations or formications but they do not have headaches. These individuals may require angiography if it is suspected that they have had a TIA.

Nonprodromal migraines include the headaches referred to as the common migraine. There are no focal deficits or warning before the headaches. The headache is unilateral. Some focal neurological deficits begin after a headache starts. This is not rare and yet not well appreciated.

Complicated migraines have a definite, prolonged focal neurological deficit. These may be visual (retinal) or unilateral trunk, arm or leg. They persist after the headache is gone (Table 5-2).

The migraine headache is unilateral, throbbing, usually frontal. A prodrome may be photophobia, scintillations, scotoma, aphasia, or unilateral symptoms. Pupillary dilation is not rare. Family history is positive in over 70 percent (Table 5-3).

Migraine treatment is either acute or prophylactic. Acute treatment is usually ergots, Midrin, or pain medications; prophylactic treatment includes Inderal, amitriptyline,[6] other beta blockers or calcium channel blockers, Cardizem.

Cluster headaches are very different. Severe, unilateral forehead pain is always in the same location and on the same side, often retro-orbital. It occurs most commonly in males, 10 to 1. These individuals wake up about an hour after they go to sleep with a severe headache lasting only a few minutes. They "just can't stand it" and cannot sit still. They do not lie down to relieve their headache as migraine patients do; they have to walk around. Unilateral redness of the eye, nasal stuffiness, or numbness often occurs. They can not drink alcohol during the cluster headaches. As per the term, cluster headaches occur for several months, then go away for a period.

Treatment is acute or prophylactic. Methylsurgide, despite the retroperitoneal fibrosis occurrence, can be very helpful. Once the cluster is past, the effort is to get the patient off the medication. Acute treatment is ergots or oxygen.

In summary, distinct characteristics help distinguish migraine from cluster: migraine goes from side to side and cluster stays on one side; almost never is there a family history in cluster, very common in migraine; also, the clinical characteristics differ (Table 5-4).

OTHER VASCULAR HEADACHES

Nonmigraine vascular headaches need to be mentioned.[7] They are hypoxic states, including carbon monoxide poisoning, the nitrites, and caffeine withdrawal. Postconcussion or post-traumatic headaches often have a vascular quality that is similar

Table 5-3. Differential Diagnosis Headache

	Frequency	Onset	Duration	Pain	Symptoms/Signs	Male/Female Distribution
Migraine	1–2/month Rarely >1/Neck	Gradual	Typically 12–18 hours	Throbbing; Unilateral; May switch sides	Nausea Visual aura	3:1 Female
Cluster	1–3/night	Sudden	½–1½ hours	Unilateral; Steady; Retro-orbital	Tearing; Horner's nasal stuffiness	10:1 Male
Muscle Contraction	Often Continuous	Gradual	8–12 hours Usual	Steady, Dull; Hatband	None	Equal
Psychogenic	Omnipresent	—	Omnipresent	Described as "Terrible"; Diffuse	None	Equal

Table 5-4. Characteristic Features Contrasting Migraine and Cluster

	Cluster	Migraine
Age onset	25–50	10–10
Sex	99% Male	65–75% Female
Occurrence of attacks	Daily for Cluster Weeks to months	Intermittent (2–8/Month)
Seasonal occurrence	Spring/Fall	No Variance
Family history	7%	90%
Number of attacks	1–6/Day	2–8/Month
Location of pain	Unilateral Periorbital	Unilateral
Duration of pain	10–180 Minutes	4–48 Hours
Prodromes	Absent	25%
Nausea	<5%	>85%
Blurred vision	Infrequent	Common
Lacrimation	Frequent	Infrequent
Nasal congestion	70%	Rare
Ptosis	30%	<2%
Miosis	50%	Absent
Polyuria	2%	40%
Activity during pain	Cannot sit still	Lie down
Relief by O_2	Yes	No

to migraine, but beginning after a head trauma.[8,9] Many of these patients, if reassured, and their physician stays with them, eventually say, "You know, it's not very bad anymore, I'm tolerating it." Postconvulsive headaches are short-lived, occurring after a seizure. The hangover headache is nondescript but frequent in our society. Hypercapnia, hypoglycemia, headache associated with elevated blood pressure, and vasomotor reaction headaches associated with nasal sinus problems may all be "vascular-like." Headaches due to inflammation of the cranial nerve structures are common from infections (basilar) or carcinomatous meningitis (Table 5-2).

Extracranial Causes of Headache

In benign intracranial hypertension (pseudotumor cerebri) the headache is diffuse and chronic, usually in young women with papilledema and visual loss. On lumbar puncture, the CSF pressure is increased. The headache is often relieved by decreasing the pressure with a spinal puncture. In these patients the concern is that visual loss may occur if they are not closely followed, besides, of course, the discomfort of the headache. Often, repeated taps are needed. If this fails, a lumboperitoneal or a ventriculoperitoneal shunt may be used.

Many of these young women have had a depressive episode within a few months before the onset of their intracranial hypertension. Associated etiologies include steroids, birth control pills, or vitamin E or A abuse. In an episode of depression, when the cortisol returns towards normal during recovery, perhaps the response to intracellular edema is altered.

Pheochromocytoma may cause headaches occurring with intermittent hypertension. Other individuals develop a headache on exertion. Initially, subarachnoid hemorrhage must always be considered. A severe headache may come on at the height of intercourse (i.e., at climax), or headache associated with cough, sneeze, or altitude may also suggest subarachnoid hemorrhage. When seen in the Emergency Room the first time, they should have a lumbar puncture or head CT scan. For example: An eighteen-year-old high school boy has been running the 100-yard dash for 2 years, but suddenly has a severe headache after running one. In the emergency room, one fears a subarachnoid hemorrhage and performs a lumbar puncture or CT scan. If he is not seen until 3 days later, is without headache and back to normal, this was probably an exertional headache. About 10 percent of individuals with exertional headache will have a structural abnormality, such as subdural hematoma, intracranial tumor, or brain abscess. These headaches are otherwise found to be benign except for the discomfort from pain.

Cerebral vascular disease causes a nonspecific headache although strokes in two locations are relatively specific. A severe frontal headache that follows backward over the vertex is almost always an anterior cerebral aneurysm rupture. Unfortunately, however, if a person says they had a sudden bad pain that has gone straight back, these are the individuals who often may go into coma within minutes to hours. The posterior cerebral artery aneurysm is almost always periorbital and behind the eye. A diabetic third nerve palsy also has headache and both cause an oculomotor cranial nerve palsy with the diabetic situation classically having spared the pupil. A posterior cerebral artery aneurysm affects the pupil, although occasionally it may be spared. Headache from other cerebral vascular disease is highly nonspecific in character or location.

Headaches occur from other extracranial causes. Temporal arteritis occurs in the fifty-five year or older patient. The headache is diffuse or may be localized to the temporal area. It is associated with jaw claudication, polymyalgia rheumatica, visual loss, fever, and other symptoms. A large temporal vessel may be palpable. The erythrocyte sedimentation rate (ESR) is almost always elevated. A normal ESR is rare but has been reported. In our biopsy-proven cases at Duke from 1970 to 1980, not one had a normal ESR.

Headache or Face Pain from Cranial Nerves

Pain from cranial nerves produces several syndromes. In trigeminal neuralgia (tic douloureux) the pain is associated with fifth nerve involvement. There is usually no sensory loss in the fifth nerve distribution. Tolosa-Hunt syndrome is pain retro-orbitally, primarily associated with other cranial nerve involvement in the superior orbital fissure. In addition to sensory loss, they have fourth and sixth nerve palsy. "Ice-cream headache" is a severe headache after one has eaten ice cream quickly. It is associated with a drop in body temperature by 1 centigrade. Possibly this is due to glosso-pharyngeal nerve stimulation.

Tic douloureux (trigeminal neuralgia) should be limited to a specific syndrome. This involves the II or III division of cranial nerve V. In about 60 percent the pain is in III and 40 percent in II and almost never in I. But the I division of cranial nerve

V is affected in herpes zoster causing neuralgia. Elderly patients may have herpes lesions on the forehead, often involving the eye. Soon afterwards, usually within weeks, they develop a painful neuralgia in the forehead called herpes zoster ophthalmacus neuralgia. They almost universally become depressed, and are difficult to treat. Tic douloureux, however, involves either division III or II unilaterally. It is more common on the right side than the left. Almost always a trigger point can be found to initiate the pain which starts medially and radiates laterally. The pain is sharp, severe, and stabbing, lasting for a few seconds, even though there may be an underlying ache. Tegretol or other anticonvulsants can treat this medically and sometimes a surgical (Janetta) procedure is required to produce relief.

Referred pain syndromes include those from the eyes, sinuses, teeth, temporomandibular joint, and the neck. Occipital neuralgia with pain from occipital nerve injury is associated with an often palpable trigger point. Neck-tongue syndrome, described in individuals with cervical spondylosis, occurs when they turn their head, producing tongue numbness and headache.

Intracranial Hemorrhage

Subarachnoid hemorrhage is a clinically important cause of severe headache. About 20 percent of subarachnoid hemorrhage patients die with the first bleed from an intracerebral aneurysm; and the second subarachnoid hemorrhage causes about 40 to 50 percent to die. Severe headache, "the worst they ever had," along with meningismus and somnolence suggests this diagnosis.

As already mentioned, arteritis is an important cause of headache. In temporal arteritis and granulomatous arteritis (or isolated cerebral vasculitis) diffuse headache is common.

Referred pain, ocular pain, and oral or nasal sinus must be remembered on the differential diagnosis of headache.

Intracerebral hemorrhage may produce a sudden severe headache, usually followed shortly by decreased level of consciousness and then hemiparesis. This is very serious because of the location of the hemorrhage and secondary swelling. If cerebellar in location, it may be a surgical emergency.

IATROGENIC HEADACHE

Hypertensive medications may cause headaches or increase preexisting symptoms. Ergot treatment is used for migraine treatment but chronic ergot usage leads to headaches, i.e., ergot poisoning. Although many people say caffeine relieves their headache—withdrawal from it can also cause headache. Some antibiotics seem to cause headaches. Fortunately, their prescription is usually limited to 10 to 14 days. Birth control pills may cause headaches and may produce vascular headaches. Basilar artery thrombosis in young women who smoke and have vascular headaches causing brain stem infarctions has been associated with migraine.

REFERENCES

1. Dalesseo DJ: *Wolfe's Headache and Other Head Pain*, 4th ed, New York, Oxford University Press, 1980.
2. Diamond S, Dalesseo DJ: *The Practicing Physician's Approach to Headache*. Baltimore, Williams & Wilkins, 1982.
3. Definition of migraine by the Research Group on Migraine and Headache. In Lance JW, *Mechanism and Management of Headache*, 4th ed Sydney, Butterworth's, 1982.
4. Sargent JD, Green EE, Walters ED: The use of autogenic feedback training in a pilot study of migraine and tension headache. *Headache* 1972; 12:120–124.
5. Budzinsky T, Stoyva J, Adler C: Feedback induced muscle relaxation application to tension headache. *Behav Ther Exper Psychol* 1970; 1:205.
6. Couch JR, Ziegler DK, Hassanein R: Amitriptyline in the prophylaxis of migraine: Effectiveness in relationship of antimigraine and antidepressant drugs. *Neurol* 1976; 26:121.
7. Classification of headache. *JAMA* 1962; 169:717–718.
8. Simon DJ, Wolff HG: Studies on headache: Mechanism of chronic post-traumatic headache. *Psychosomatic Med* 1946; 8:227.
9. Kelly M: Headaches: Traumatic and rheumatic. The cervical somatic lesion. *Med J Aust* 1942; 2:479.

Chapter 6

TEMPOROMANDIBULAR JOINT DISORDERS

Diagnosis and Treatment

Edward A. Dolan, D.D.S.

INTRODUCTION

Craniofacial pain is encountered frequently in everyday practice. A logical and thorough approach to the patient's problem utilizing a multidisciplinary team approach is beneficial. The clinician should keep an open mind in the diagnostic process so that an accurate patient assessment can be made.

Due to difficulties in diagnosing the particular etiology, temporomandibular joint disorders are a perplexing problem to most clinicians. There is a vast amount of literature on the clinical treatments for a patient with temporomandibular joint problems, but unfortunately many of these treatment modalities were based upon interpretations of clinical findings and not upon sound working diagnoses. This has led to a wide variation in treatment methods which are derived from interpretation of inaccurate clinical information. A complete understanding of the classification, separation, and interrelationship between the various functional and structural disorders is necessary. Too often, we, as clinicians, diagnose our patient as having TMJ without performing a thorough diagnostic evaluation and arriving at an accurate differential diagnosis. Both functional and structural disorders of the temporomandibular joint can mimic other neurological disorders, and it is not uncommon therefore to find a temporomandibular joint patient who presents with an underlying misdiagnosed neurological problem. Only after a sound working diagnosis has been formulated can effective therapy be rendered, whether invasive or noninvasive. Evaluation from a variety of health professionals—oral and maxillofacial surgeon, orthodontist, general dentist, and psychiatrist or psychologist—should be obtained. Therefore it is the clinician's responsibility to be well versed in the differential diagnosis of various craniofacial pain syndromes that may coexist in the temporomandibular joint patient.

There is an increasing need for a thorough evaluation of our diagnostic and treatment methods and a standardized method of classifying, diagnosing, and treating temporomandibular joint problems. These standards can be realized with continuing sound scientific and clinical research. In addition, it is important that this information be disseminated to all health professionals involved in this treatment.

Anatomy

The temporomandibular joint is a diarthrodial joint (ginglymoarthrodial) formed by the temporal bone and the mandibular condyle (Figure 6-1). The condylar surface is covered by dense avascular fibrous tissue and articulates with the glenoid fossa and the temporal bone. The condyle measures 8 to 10 mm in an anterior posterior direction and is convex in shape, while in a medial to lateral direction it measures 10 to 15 mm and is concave in appearance. It forms by endochondral ossification and is the only true joint of the skull with the exception of the auditory ossicles. The condyle articulates principally with the glenoid fossa and the articular eminence. These articular surfaces consist of three areas: the preglenoid slope, the entoglenoid process, and the articular eminence. The articular eminence or tubercle is a nonarticulating surface and serves as the attachment for the lateral ligament. There are three ligaments associated

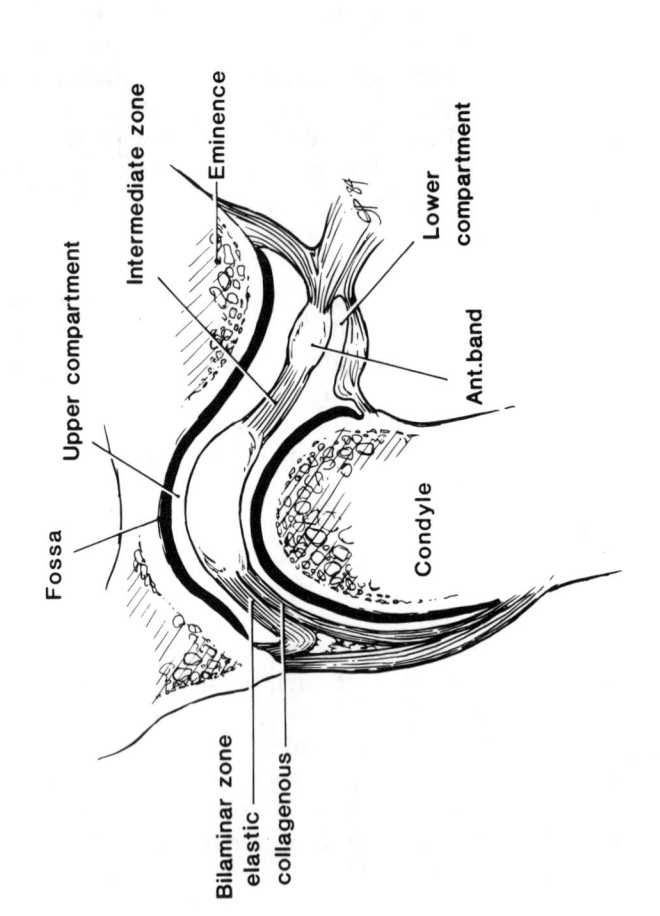

Figure 6-1. Sagittal view of normal TMJ anatomy.

with the temporomandibular joint, one intrinsic and two accessory. The two accessory ligaments, the sphenomandibular and stylomandibular, only function to limit maximum opening in a vertical and protrusive direction and, therefore, do not influence movement directly. The temporomandibular ligament does influence the movement of the joint and also strengthens the lateral surface of the joint capsule. It is composed of two bands: a superficial band inferiorly and posteriorly which supports the condyle in a vertical direction, and the medial or horizontal band which begins at the crest of the articular tubercle and runs posteriorly attaching with the disk on the lateral surface of the condyle.

There are many muscles in the head and neck which influence temporomandibular joint function. The external pterygoid muscles, however, affect the joint most directly. The muscle is composed of two bellies (superior and inferior) which function antagonistically. The superior portion is smaller, functions during closure, and serves to support the elastic fibers of the meniscus. This provides stabilization and counteracts the tension of the elastic fiber posteriorly. The inferior belly is larger and functions during mandibular opening.

The arterial supply is from branches of the external carotid artery. The superficial temporal and maxillary arteries provide nutrition posteriorly, while the internal maxillary via the masseteric artery supplies the anterior portion of the joint capsule.

The main source of innervation to the temporomandibular joint is from the auriculotemporal nerve. This nerve supplies the posterior, lateral, and anterolateral portions of the joint, while the masseteric nerve supplies the anteromedial and the posterior deep temporal innervates the medial surface. The innervation to the joint conforms to Hilton's Law, which states that the skin and muscles overlying the joint are supplied by the same nerve root that supplies the joint itself. This fact makes differential diagnosis of intrinsic joint pain difficult, particularly in the patient with both a functional and structural disorder.

The capsule of the temporomandibular joint is composed of collagen fibers which are not under tension. The capsule is well organized and extends from the tympanic plate to the condylar neck. It is supported laterally by the temporomandibular ligament which strengthens and supports the capsule. The anterior portion of the meniscus and capsule are fused, with the capsule possessing a copious innervation. There is no capsule found on the medial or lateral one-half of the anterior aspect of the joint, only loose connective tissue. This is often known as the Achilles heel of the TMJ.

The meniscus of the joint is composed of dense fibrous collagen and divides the joint into an upper and lower joint space. In the newborn, the meniscus is vascular but becomes avascular between the ages of three and five. The disk divides the joint into an upper and lower joint space, varies in shape, and measures 2 to 4 mm centrally. The meniscus attaches to the capsule anteriorly and ends in the retrodistal pad posteriorly. On the lateral and medial portions it is attached to the poles of the condyle, but not to the capsule.

Posteriorly, the bilaminar zone of the meniscus is composed of three strata: 1) the superior, made of elastin and attached to the tympanic plate, 2) the middle posterior, composed of areolar tissue, and 3) the inferior strata composed of collagen. Anteriorly, the bilaminar zone is attached to the external pterygoid muscle and is quite vascular, as is the portion just anterior to the bilaminar zone.

Physiology

Functionally, the temporomandibular joints act as a unit by virtue of being connected by the mandible, the only movable bone of the skull. Intricate coordination by the muscles of mastication produce its various movements. The parotid gland, which overlies the masseter muscle, extends behind the ramus of the mandible between it and the external auditory meatus. This prohibits the mandible from moving in only a hinge motion and necessitates that a gliding motion be used. The simple hinge action, which is the initial movement, occurs in the lower joint space, while the gliding motion takes place in the upper joint space.

Depression and Elevation

During both depression and elevation there is a combination of translation and rotational movement. Initially, when depression occurs, the movement is primarily hinge or rotatory, then as opening continues there is a combination of both the hinge and gliding movements. Depression is primarily accomplished by the external pterygoid muscle with assistance by the geniohyoid, mylohyoid, and digastric muscles.

Closing of the mandible is accomplished principally by the masseteric, medial pterygoid, and temporalis muscles and is translatory in nature. As closing occurs there is again a combination of both rotary and translatory movement as the mandible completes its closure.

Protrusion and Retrusion

Protrusion of the mandible occurs by the action of the medial pterygoid muscles. As the mandible is moved forward the condyle and articular disks are also pulled forward, and since this is a gliding motion it takes place in the upper compartment. Retrusion of the mandible is also translatory and is performed by the temporalis and suprahyoid muscles. Most individuals' retrusive movements are limited and seldom more than 2 mm.

Lateral Shift

Right and left lateral excursions of the mandible are made by the external pterygoid muscle. The side toward which the mandible moves is called the working side and the opposite side is called the balancing side. On the working side the condyle makes a slight rotation about a vertical axis accompanied by a slight lateral shift in the direction of the movement. This minimal downward, forward, and lateral movement is called the Bennett movement. The balancing side undergoes a downward, forward, and inward movement and, therefore, assumes the greatest stress during function. All mandibular movements depend on the interrelationship of the dentition, position of the condyle in the fossa, and the interdigitation of the dentition if muscle coordination is to be smooth and free of interference.

CLASSIFICATION OF TEMPOROMANDIBULAR JOINT DISORDERS

Temporomandibular joint disorders have been classified by several methods. The classification in Table 6-1 was published by the American Academy of Craniomandibular Disorders.[1] Often, whether the etiology is functional or structural, the symptoms are similar. Complaints of headache, earache, clicking and popping, grating, and limitation of movement are common. The

Table 6-1. Classification of Craniomandibular Disorders*

I. Craniomandibular Disorders of Organic Origin
   A. Articular disturbances
      1. Disc derangements
      2. Condylar displacement
      3. Inflammatory conditions
      4. Arthritis
      5. Ankylosis
      6. Fractures
      7. Neoplasia
      8. Developmental abnormalities
   B. Nonarticular disturbances
      1. Neuromuscular conditions
      2. Occlusal conditions
II. Craniomandibular Disorders of Nonorganic Origin
   A. Myofascial pain dysfunction syndrome
   B. Chronic craniofacial and cervical pains
   C. Phantom pains
   D. Positive occlusal sense
   E. Conversion hysteria
III. Craniomandibular disorders of nonorganic origin combined with secondary organic tissue changes

*Adapted from McNeill C et al: Craniomandibular (TMJ) disorders—The state of the art. *J Prosthet Dent* 1980; 44:434.

clinician must determine if the etiology is primarily functional, structural, or a combination of both.

It is imperative that the clinician appreciate this classification in order to accurately assess the patient's temporomandibular joint disorder, formulate an accurate differential diagnosis, and provide sequential treatment. It is beyond the scope of this chapter to cover all the classifications; the most pertinent regarding temporomandibular joint disorders will be reviewed.

PATIENT EVALUATION

Diagnosis of the patient with a temporomandibular joint disorder requires that a thorough history be obtained. During the history taking it is important to distinguish between complaints of pain and complaints of dysfunction. An example of a useful temporomandibular joint questionnaire which may be used is seen in Figure 6-2.

Figure 6-2
Temporomandibular Joint Questionnaire

1. Name
   Age
2. Medical History (past and current).
3. Dental History (past and current).
4. Have you been previously treated for this problem?
5. Do you have pain?
6. Is the pain in the temple, ear, or jaw?
7. Is there pain in the right, left, or both joints?
8. Is the pain sharp, dull, and how long does it last?
9. Do you have headaches?
10. Do you have any history of trauma?
11. Do you have and back, neck, or shoulder pain?
12. Do you clench your teeth during the day?
13. Do you grind your teeth at night?
14. Is there any clicking, popping, or grating when you open and close your mouth?
15. Does your jaw lock open or closed?
16. Do you have history of emotional or psychiatric problems?

Clinical examination should again be directed at distinguishing between a functional or structural disorder. A dental examination emphasizing the relationship of the dentition should be noted. Soft tissue examination should be directed at the muscles of the head and neck; palpation of these muscles may elicit any tenderness. Measurement of mandibular opening should be done, giving special attention to any pain or asymmetrical movements, and palpation and auscultation of the condylar heads may reveal clicking, popping, or grating. Finally, a neurologic evaluation of the patient must be performed to determine if other pain syndromes are present.

Laboratory evaluations are indicated if there is a suspicion of a systemic etiology, or to aid in differential diagnosis. A complete blood count with differential should be performed. In addition, an erythrocyte sedimentation rate, a rheumatoid factor, and latex fixation test may be utilized. A study of a joint aspiration can be done in order to determine if gout or infection exists.

Radiographic evaluation should be performed as part of the initial examination. A Panorex and lateral transcranial radiographs will be useful aids in order to determine if structural damage is present. The lateral transcranial radiograph is the most common and can be used to assess joint space and condylar contour, position, and excursion. More sophisticated radiographs such as transmaxillary and transpharyngeal projection are seldom needed. Tomography is very useful when an arthritic condition is suspected. If internal derangements (disk abnormalities) are diagnosed, then arthrography or computerized axial tomography should be utilized.

ARTICULAR DISTURBANCES

Degenerative Joint Disease

Degenerative joint disease of the temporomandibular joint occurs secondary to overloading of the joint itself.[2,3] Early signs of this functional overloading may be spasm of the masticatory muscles or stiffness or locking of the jaw with accompanied clicking and popping. The etiology of this overloading can frequently be traced to a parafunctional habit such as clenching or grinding of the teeth, or loss of posterior tooth support which may contribute to misplaced directional forces and excessive overloading. The condition is usually unilateral; however, it is not uncommon for the disease to be bilateral. Most patients present with symptoms greater than 9 months in duration, which gradually subside over the next 2 years. The initial reaction is muscular dysfunction and is expressed as joint clicking with mandibular deviation. As the disease process becomes more advanced, osteophyte formation causes perforation of the meniscus and increased dysfunction.

Clinically, the patient presents with a history of pain which has been nonresponsive to conservative treatment. Women are affected more than men, usually in the third to fourth decade. The pain is well localized, insidious in onset, and there is usually a history of trauma. Muscle splinting, uncoordinated jaw movements, crepitation and grating within the joint itself are seen.

The degenerative process begins within the cartilaginous matrix of the articular cartilage, progressing to the subcondylar core, and finally to the joint capsule. Histopathologically the disease progresses through four stages: 1) fibrillation (loss of collagen cohesion), denudation and eburnation (mineralization and loss of fibrous surface), 2) perforation and microfracture of bony endplates with complete collapse of articular surface, 3) erosion and replacement of fibrous tissue, and 4) repair of bony plates. Radiographically, one sees joint space narrowing, peripheral osteophyte formation, decreased range of motion, and flattening of the condylar head.

Rheumatoid Arthritis

Rheumatoid arthritis affects women more frequently than men between the ages of twenty-five and fifty-five.[4] Two-thirds of all patients with rheumatoid arthritis show temporomandibular joint symptoms. The patient usually reports feeling generally ill, with fatigue, fever, weight loss, and pain and stiffness in the joints. Later in the disease a polyarthritis develops in which the smaller joints are affected and subcutaneous nodules and vascular lesions appear.

On clinical examination the patients present with deep dull pain in the preauricular area, and ear complaints are common. In advanced cases, loss of vertical dimension may lead to a malocclusion. Palpation of the temporomandibular joints also demonstrates crepitus and grating as degeneration of the joint structures progresses.

In contrast to degenerative joint disease, rheumatoid arthritis is a primary disease of the joint capsule, and inflammatory in nature. The disease process itself consists of two stages, the first involving a systemic inflammatory process which precipitates joint inflammation, and the second involving an autoimmune reaction to antigens produced by the initial inflammation. As progression from the acute inflammatory states to more chronic granulomatous formation occurs, bony erosion of the condylar head with osteophyte formation is seen. Radiographically there is a characteristic cloudy hazy joint space which is narrowed, and the condyle is sharp in appearance.

Treatment of both disease processes should be aimed at palliation, beginning with conservative treatment, and then advancing to more invasive procedures. Nonsteroidal anti-inflammatory drugs or aspirin help reduce inflammation and provide analgesia. Physical therapy utilizing ultrasound, moist heat, and restricting mandibular movement also may be useful. Intraarticular injections of steroids are not indicated in these patients, since multiple steroid injections lead to an acceleration of the degenerative process through chemical remodeling.[5] If conservative measures are not effective, consideration should be given to surgical treatment.

Surgical criteria should be based upon persistent pain, radiographic changes and, above all, an accurate differential diagnosis. The most common surgical treatment is the high condylectomy (condylar shave). This procedure removes the irregularities of the articular surface of the condyle, and thereby recontours the condylar head. Repair or replacement of the meniscus may be indicated, depending on the extent of the degenerative process. If the meniscus must be removed, then replacement with some alloplastic material such as a silastic or proplast Teflon implant should be done. Following surgical treatment, aggressive physical therapy, particularly jaw-opening exercises and ultrasound therapy should be instituted.

Hypermobility

Hypermobility of the temporomandibular joint occurs when the condyle translates anterior to the articular eminence. The condition may be self-reducing (subluxation) or non-self reducing (dislocation).[6] In dislocation the patient usually requires manual reduction in order to return the condyle to the fossa, while in subluxation cases this is not necessary.

Increased mobility is commonly a result of muscle spasm which produces increased capsular laxity and meniscus dysfunction. Phenothiazine derivative, psychological problems, or rare conditions such as Ehlers-Danlos or Marfan's syndrome may be the cause.

Initial treatment of the acute emergency is palliative and consists of such things as reduction of the dislocation, sedation with Valium or Demerol, and intermaxillary fixation. If it is determined that this is a chronic condition, consideration should be given to surgical treatment.

There have been a variety of surgical procedures to correct this problem, but the most common is temporomandibular joint eminectomy.[5] Removal of the entire eminence permits good condylar translation in an anterior direction and eliminates dislocation of the condyle anterior to the eminence.

Hypomobility

Hypomobility of the temporomandibular joint may be classified into two categories; true ankylosis or false ankylosis.[7] True ankylosis is a bony or fibrous fusion of the articular surface of the condyle and glenoid fossa. In 50 percent of the cases, trauma is the predominant etiology; however, infection, inflammation, or birth injury may be the cause. Histologically, there is degeneration of the meniscus with narrowing of the joint space. Cartilage destruction and fibrous replacement leads to eventual joint fusion. Clinically the patient with a unilateral ankylosis may have a facial asymmetry with fullness on the affected side. If the ankylosis is bilateral, then an open bite deformity may exist. Pain is usually minimal to nonexistent in the patient with true bony ankylosis. Radiographically there is a cloudy narrow joint space, which is best seen using lateral tomography. Treatment usually consists of a condylectomy in conjunction with an interpositional implant in patients with a fibrous ankylosis. In true bony ankylosis, a gap arthroplasty with an interpositional implant material is the procedure of choice and a coronoidectomy is almost always performed. Interpositional materials may be biologic such as fascia, cartilage, or dermis, or alloplastic, such as silicone rubber or proplast Teflon sheeting. In children, particularly before puberty, costochondral or metatarsal grafts are used to allow symmetrical growth of the mandible. If the bony ankylosis is very extensive, complete replacement of the condylar process and fossa may need to be done with a proplast coated Vitalium prosthesis.

False ankylosis may be myogenic, neurogenic, or psychogenic in origin. The most common etiology is muscle trismus associated with infection, trauma, or surgery. Restriction or impingement of the coronoid process of the mandible secondary to facial fractures may result in a fibrous union to the zygomatic arch. Iatrogenic causes may be produced by dental surgery or injection of the temporomandibular joint leading to fibrosis. Treatment includes coronoidectomy and excision of fibrous adhesions along the muscle pathways.

Internal Derangements (Disk Abnormalities)

Internal derangements of the temporomandibular joint may be characterized by an abnormal relationship between the disk, condyle, and fossa.[8] The primary etiology of the internal derangement appears to be traumatic in origin. The elastic and collagenous portions of the bilaminar zone become stretched and redundant, thereby producing this abnormal condyle disk relationship. If this continues, complete degeneration of the meniscus and perforation will occur. The disk abnormalities may be classified into three categories: subluxated (self-reducing),

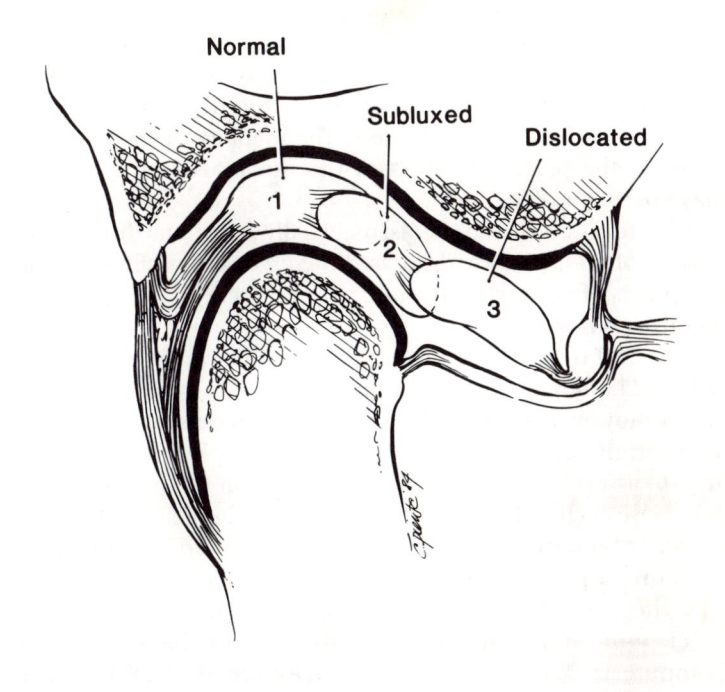

Figure 6-3. Schematic illustration of a normal, subluxated, and dislocated TMJ meniscus.

dislocated (nonreducing), or perforated meniscus (Figure 6-3).

Subluxation of the meniscus or anterior displacement with reduction is often characterized by reciprocal clicking. As the jaw opens, clicking occurs as a result of condylar movement across the junction of the bilaminar zone and meniscus; this returns the condyle to the meniscus. On closing, the condyle slips posterior to the meniscus, producing a closing click, and again the meniscus is anteriorly displaced. Clinically the patient has pain and deviation toward the affected side; clicking and popping are heard on opening and closing.

Anterior displacement of the meniscus without reduction is

termed closed lock. In this condition the meniscus is completely dislocated and the condyle cannot translate the junction of the bilaminar zone and meniscus. Patients have difficulty achieving maximum opening, and deviation to the affected side occurs. There is no clicking heard due to the inability of the condyle to translate the posterior aspect of the meniscus and the patients may complain of pain.

Perforation of the meniscus usually occurs in the posterior portion of an anteriorly dislocated meniscus. Clinically the patient complains of pain, clicking, and popping; crepitus is evident on the affected side.

Lateral transcranial or panoramic radiographs do not demonstrate bony changes in the early stages of internal derangements; however, in chronic dislocation or meniscus perforation, degenerative changes may occur. Arthrography is therefore utilized to assess the position of the meniscus in relation to the condyle.[9] Dye such as Renografin 60 is injected into either the upper, lower, or both joint spaces; this may be followed by tomography or fluoroscopy. Fluoroscopy enables the clinician to observe not only the position and condition of the meniscus, but also the exact point at which the meniscus reduces during function. Computerized tomography has been extremely useful in the diagnosis of internal derangements. Its main advantage is that it is a noninvasive procedure and provides a direct image of the meniscus. The disadvantages are the inability to evaluate the joint under function and the cost factor.

Treatment of internal derangement is aimed at repositioning the condyle and meniscus into a functional position. Conservative treatment utilizing anterior positioning splints, which position the condyle anteriorly on the meniscus, may be used initially. Adjustment of the splint over an 8 to 12 week period is aimed at maintaining the condyle in its most posterior position while providing a good functional relationship. If nonsurgical treatment does not provide correction, then surgical treatment may be indicated. Diagnosis is established utilizing computerized tomography or arthrotomography. Surgical treatment again is aimed at providing a good condyle meniscus relationship. A wedge meniscoplasty procedure is used and is accomplished by removing a small portion of the redundant tissue in the posterior attachment of the meniscus and then surgically reattaching the meniscus into the proper position. If the meniscus cannot be repositioned or is degenerated beyond repair, then a menisectomy, arthroplasty, and insertion of an implant material should be performed. Postoperatively, the patients are placed on aggressive physical therapy treatments consisting of active and passive jaw exercises and ultrasound therapy.

Myofascial Pain Dysfunction Syndrome (MPD Syndrome)

Monson, in 1920, proposed that noise in the middle ear coupled with deafness and lack of concentration was secondary to pressure produced by the mandibular condyle on certain nerves.[10] Decker also proposed a direct connection between ear pain and the temporomandibular joint.[11] In 1934, Costen, an otolaryngologist, related the clinical symptoms of burning tongue, ringing in the ears, and hearing loss to overclosure of the mandible which resulted in pressure on nerve fibers.[12] He proposed that these symptoms were directly related to a decrease in vertical dimension of occlusion and thereby shifted the emphasis to malocclusion of the dentition. In the 1950s, Sicher, an anatomist, disproved this earlier theory of Costen by demonstrating that there was no anatomical correlation between these symptoms and condylar pressure on the articular nerves.[13] They felt that the neuromuscular system rather than the temporomandibular joint articulation was the etiology of these disorders. In 1969, Laskin elaborated on the earlier work of Sicher and Schwartz and popularized the "psychophysiologic theory" of the myofascial pain dysfunction syndrome illustrating very well the various signs and symptoms of myofascial pain.[14] It was at this time that the well-known condition of "temporomandibular joint syndrome" was renamed "myofascial pain dysfunction syndrome."

Four popular theories have been proposed as to the etiology of myofascial pain dysfunction syndrome. The mechanical displacement theory of Monson, Costen, and Prentiss theorized that condylar position as the initiating factor in this syndrome.[10,12,15] Following this, the muscle theory came into vogue. Proponents of this theory felt that stress, tension, and anxiety affected the jaw musculature. It was also thought that any uncoordinated jaw movements resulting from malocclusion, muscle fatigue, or any dysfunction in the normal chewing pattern could be causative.

The neuromuscular theory stated that the increase in muscle tone, which was seen clinically, was a direct result of a functional imbalance between the occlusion and the temporomandibular joint. It was also stated that a history of stress, tension, and anxiety were factors. Therefore, any interference in the relationship of the dentition can cause a grinding or clenching of the teeth which in turn produces muscle spasm and, finally, pain.

The psychophysiologic theory according to Laskin (Figure 6-4) states that extension or excessive contraction of the masticatory muscles is the prime factor and leads to muscle fatigue.[14] These muscle spasms may be a result of inadequate dental restorations, loss of posterior teeth or, more often, caused by oral habits such as clenching or grinding of the teeth.

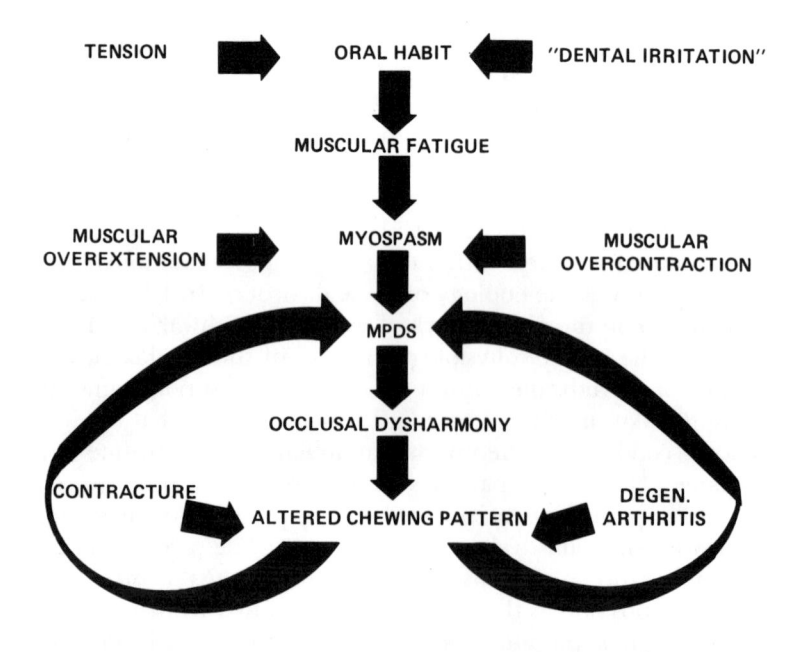

Figure 6-4. Laskin's psychophysiologic theory.

Signs and Symptoms

An accurate differential diagnosis based on correlation of the clinical and radiographic findings is essential. Separation of the extrinsic (inorganic) from the intrinsic (organic) disorders is paramount. Myofascial pain dysfunction syndrome is due to a disruption of function rather than structure. However, chronic functional problems may eventually produce organic changes within the joint itself. For example, organic changes may present themselves as internal derangements of the meniscus, accompanied by osteoarthritic changes, which result from constant overloading of the joints by altered chewing patterns and parafunctional habits.

The majority of patients (80 to 90 percent) affected are women under forty years of age. Patients usually present with dull diffuse unilateral pain in front of the ear, muscle tenderness, popping and clicking in the joint itself, and limitation of jaw function. Pain in the muscles and joint is the most common factor and often associated with headaches. The pain is relatively constant, often found to be present on arising in the morning and gradually worsening as the day progresses. The next most common complaint is muscle tenderness. This can be elicited by palpation of the masticatory muscles, particularly in the mandibular angle and temporal crest area. Palpation of the joint itself through the external auditory meatus does not produce tenderness.

The classical myofascial pain dysfunction syndrome patient usually does not present with radiographic evidence of structural changes in the temporomandibular joint. Although organic changes are not seen because the origin is basically neuromuscular, radiographs should be taken in order that all clinical data can be correlated. Radiographic survey by lateral transcranial views, in both the open and closed position, are the most useful. Diagnosis of bony pathology, condylar position, and adequacy of joint space can be obtained by these radiographs.

Treatment

A broad range of treatment has been recommended, depending on the clinician, for a patient with a diagnosed myofascial pain dysfunction syndrome, and therefore it is essential that a multidisciplinary team approach be utilized. Patient education with a clear understanding of the difference between the neuromuscular disorder of myofascial pain dysfunction syndrome and intrinsic organic disorders of the temporomandibular joint is vital. It also must be explained that both the extrinsic and intrinsic disorders of the temporomandibular joint may exist either independently or in conjunction with one another. A careful explanation of the differences in etiologies, clinical findings, and treatment methods will lead to better patient cooperation, which is absolutely necessary ry if a successful result is to be achieved. Many of these patients, whether their disorder originated extrinsically or intrinsically, have been misdiagnosed or undiagnosed. They have consulted a myriad of health professionals without relief from their pain. Patients with pain longer than 6 months have a significant amount of emotional overlay, particularly depression.[16] Extensive counseling and reassurance is often necessary at the initial visit in order to obtain good patient rapport.

Following the collection of diagnostic data and formulation of an accurate differential diagnosis, treatment is initiated. The treatment modalities are aimed at both treatment and diagnosis. Much of the initial treatment is noninvasive and reversible and always aimed at differentiating neuromuscular disorders from the true structural disorders.

Symptomatic treatment consisting of a soft diet, jaw rest, drugs, and physiotherapy is encouraged, and aids in gaining patient confidence. The only restriction in the soft diet is that of texture as all foods must be soft enough or finely minced in order to minimize chewing. Special attention should be given to maintaining adequate nutritional balance during the soft diet since many soft foods are predominantly carbohydrates.

Jaw movement limitations should be placed upon the normal functions of mastication, as well as upon other parafunctional overloading. Patients who sing, play musical instruments, and smoke pipes may need to curtail these activities. Destructive habits of clenching, bruxism, and grinding of the teeth must be minimized.

Drug therapy consisting of analgesics, muscle relaxants, anti-inflammatory agents, and local anesthesia may be used. Aspirin, because of its combined analgesic and anti-inflammatory properties, is an excellent choice for the symptomatic treatment of the myofascial pain dysfunction syndrome patient. Enteric-coated tablets may be beneficial, particularly if the buffered preparations cannot be used. Muscle relaxants, principally diazepam (5 mg as necessary for relaxation) is an excellent choice not only because of its muscle relaxant properties, but also because of its anxiolytic effects. Anti-inflammatory agents, particularly in patients who demonstrate intrinsic structural changes from conditions such as osteoarthritis or rheumatoid arthritis, are advantageous in the myofascial pain dysfunction patient. Drugs such as ibuprofen (300-600 mg every 8 hours) provide relief. If the patient is experiencing significant disability secondary to muscle spasm, a local anesthetic such as Xylocaine injected into the spastic muscle may relieve the pain and spasm.

Physiotherapy, self-administered at home and under the supervision of a physical therapist, is helpful. Moist heat compresses applied for 20 to 30 minutes are effective means of decreasing muscle hyperactivity and thereby decreased muscle tension. Heat also increases the permeability of cell membranes which promotes increased circulation to the affected area. The most commonly used methods are dry heating packs and pads or moist application with towels and washcloths. These heat applications may be used in combination with cold applications for 30 to 60 seconds, followed by another 10 to 20 minutes of moist heat. Cold application works by three methods: (1) by controlling thermal stimuli, (2) by raising the pain threshold of the skin, and (3) by decreasing histamine levels.

Multidisciplinary Approach

Behavior modification is the most useful tool for the treatment of patients with neuromuscular conditions such as myofascial pain syndrome. Biofeedback therapy in conjunction with behavioral assessment of the patient is the basis for sound treatment whether the neuromuscular condition exists alone or in combination with an intrinsic disorder. Developed in the 1960s in order to reduce stress and tension, biofeedback has had broad application in health care.[17] The therapy itself makes the patient aware of muscle tension and its relation to stress, tension, and anxiety. The patients essentially treat themselves by this method by directly controlling their stress levels. Budzynski and others were the first to employ electromyographic biofeedback induced muscle relaxation in the treatment of tension headaches.[18]

Surface electromyographic electrodes are placed on the affected muscles. The patient is educated in the role of stress, tension, and anxiety and its effect on the musculature of the head and neck. The muscle tension is then monitored via the electrodes and this information is fed back to the patient by using an electrical meter or audio signal (Figure 6-5). By utilizing this method the patient learns to control his stress voluntarily. The patient learns to consciously control neuromuscular overloading, thereby decreasing the destructive forces on the articular structures of the temporomandibular joint.

In conjunction with biofeedback therapy, it has been shown that behavioral coping skills are very beneficial in the treatment of myofascial pain. Evidence exists that demonstrates the effectiveness of teaching coping skills in order to help individuals deal with situational problems and interpersonal reactions.[19] Pain coping skill training can be incorporated, teaching patients strategies such as goal setting, imagery, distraction, and relaxation to deal with their pain.[20]

Transcutaneous electrical nerve stimulation (TENS) has been used extensively for the management of acute and chronic pain syndromes.[21,22,23] Many of the transcutaneous nerve stimulators are portable and can be worn by the patient. The units are usually single (two electrodes) or dual (four electrodes) channel models. The units maintain a constant current when connected to the skin. The pulse generator produces a low power pulsating current (10-40 MA at a rate of 20 to 200 pulses per second, given for a 30 to 60 minute period on a daily basis). This neuroelectrical stimulation intercepts the transmission of pain information to conscious levels by transmitting the electrical input from the TENS unit through large diameter afferent nerve fibers, thus not permitting smaller diameter afferent fibers to transmit pain.[24] The patient may feel a mild tingling sensation, with the pain relief lasting from one to several hours.

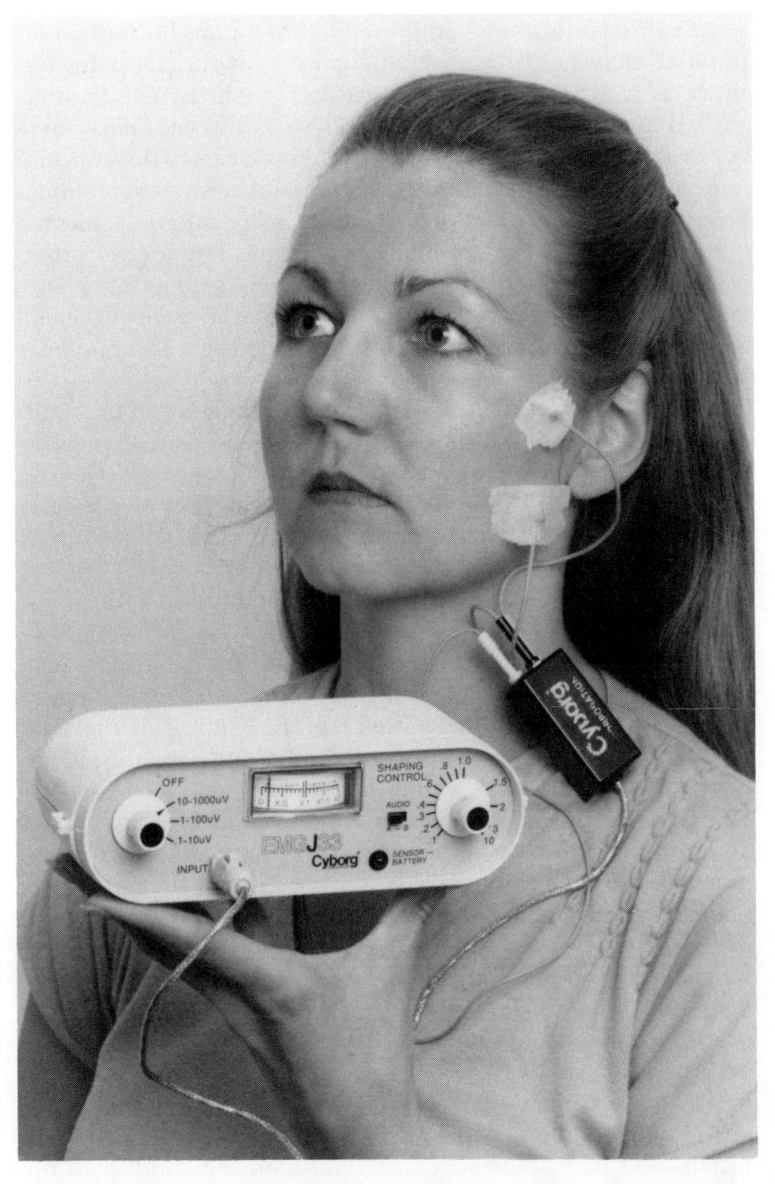

Figure 6-5. Biofeedback surface, electromyographic electrodes applied to the affected muscles.

Occlusal adjustment and disengagement has been the most popular treatment for the patient with myofascial pain dysfunction syndrome. This is because occlusal disharmony was regarded by most dentists as the etiology of this condition. There are two groups of dental clinicians who subscribe to this concept: one group believes symptoms of pain and dysfunction should be relieved prior to occlusal adjustment, while others correct the occlusion as their primary mode of therapy. The former group also feels that the use of intraoral appliances, such as bite planes and occlusal splints, are necessary treatment in order to obtain correct jaw relationship and therefore establish neuromuscular balance of the mandible.

Splint therapy in general can be a good diagnostic and treatment modality in patients with either an extrinsic or intrinsic dysfunction of the temporomandibular joint. Although their use does not usually provide definitive treatment, they are, in most instances, a very useful adjunct in patients with myofascial pain dysfunction n and related disorders.

Intraoral appliances are the most often used treatments for patients with myofascial pain dysfunction. The main objective of these appliances is to modify parafunctional habits such as the clenching, grinding, and bruxism of teeth, or to reduce muscle hyperactivity. In addition, severe loading of the temporomandibular joints is prevented. The appliance itself has many designs with such names as the Sned, Hawley, Gelb, or Shore.[25,26,27,28] These appliances may be fitted to either the upper jaw, lower jaw, or both, and can be constructed of metal, plastic, or rubber. The treatment objectives vary with the appliance. Some clinicians use appliances simply to relieve symptoms, while others have regarded them as both a diagnostic and treatment modality. Diagnostic splints therefore can be used to confirm a diagnosis of a neuromuscular disorder such as myofascial pain dysfunction syndrome and separate this condition from a simple occlusal disharmony. These splints were usually flat in design, having as their main objective to eliminate all occlusal interferences between the maxillary and mandibular teeth. Other clinicians feel that appliances that reposition the condyle in the fossa, thereby decreasing joint overload, are beneficial.

Diagnosis of specific structural alterations such as internal derangements of the temporomandibular joint in conjunction with the neuromuscular disorder requires a specific type of mandibular repositioning orthopedic appliance. There are many designs for this appliance; however, the main objective is the same: to reposition the condyle in relation to the meniscus and thereby improve the function of the articular structures.

Occlusal appliances are aimed at modification of parafunctional habits such as nocturnal bruxism. These appliances not only alter proprioceptive input from the teeth to the musculature, but also make the patient more aware of his habit by jaw repositioning. These bruxism appliances are made of a soft vinyl material and cover the entire maxillary or mandibular arch (Figure 6-6). The bite guard should be worn constantly, except during meals, while the patient is symptomatic. After the symptoms improve the appliance may be worn only at night, thus allowing the patient to maintain control of unconscious nocturnal habits and prevent a recurrence of neuromuscular symptoms. Rugh and Solberg investigated full arch maxillary splint therapy on patients with nocturnal bruxism.[29] Muscular response before, during, and after splint therapy was evaluated and indicated that nocturnal bruxism may be reduced by this splint therapy; however, there was no lasting effect, as was evidenced by the return of the nocturnal electromyographic activity to pre-treatment levels.

Physical therapy performed under the direction of a trained licensed physical therapist is important in rebuilding damaged tissues. In addition to heat and ice applications which were used initially, myotherapy is of benefit. Myotherapy, aimed at decreasing muscle spasm by retrusion reflex relaxation exercises, has produced good results. This therapy is based on the fact that when one muscle contracts there is a simultaneous reflex relaxation of the antagonist muscle (Figure 6-7).

Treatment of muscle spasms, particularly the medial and lateral pterygoids, require microwave or ultrasound diathermy. Deep heating of the muscles can be accomplished to a depth of 4 to 5 cm. If therapeutic results are not noted after 10 days, therapy should be discontinued. Galvanic stimulation by means of a electrogalvanic stimulator (Figure 6-8) produces muscle activity in those muscles which are refractory by stimulating either

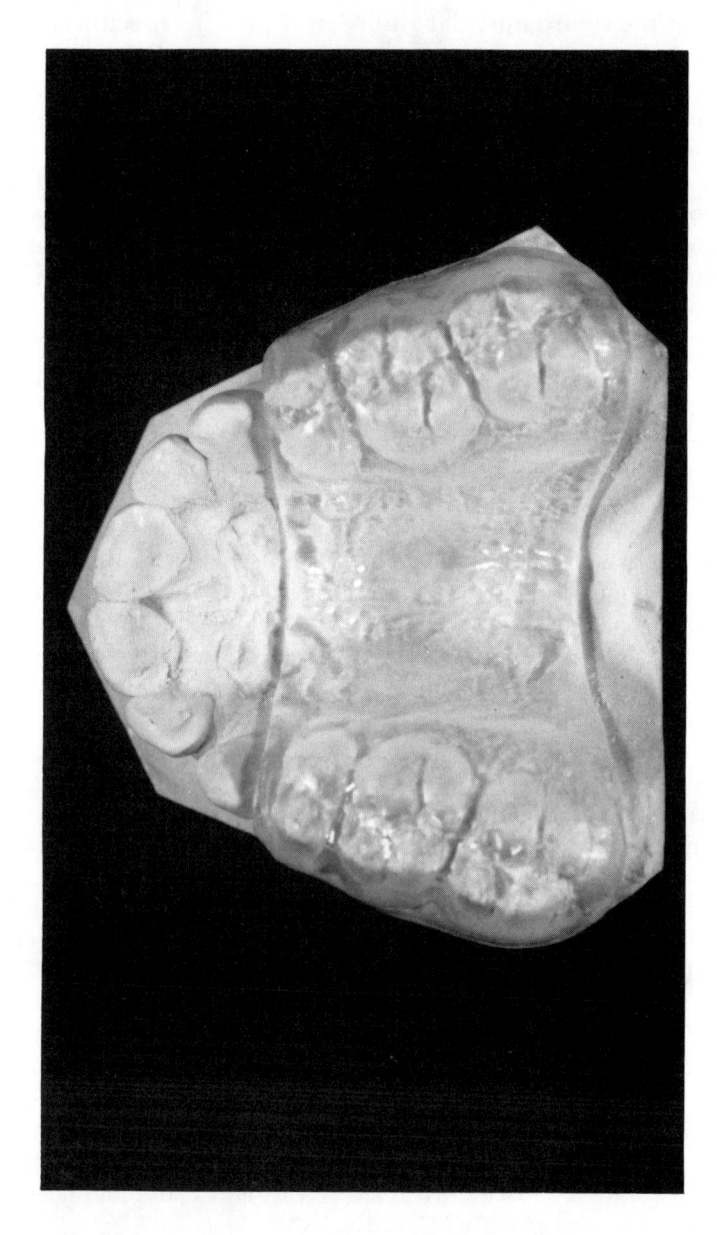

Figure 6-6. A superior view of a maxillary posterior bite guard.

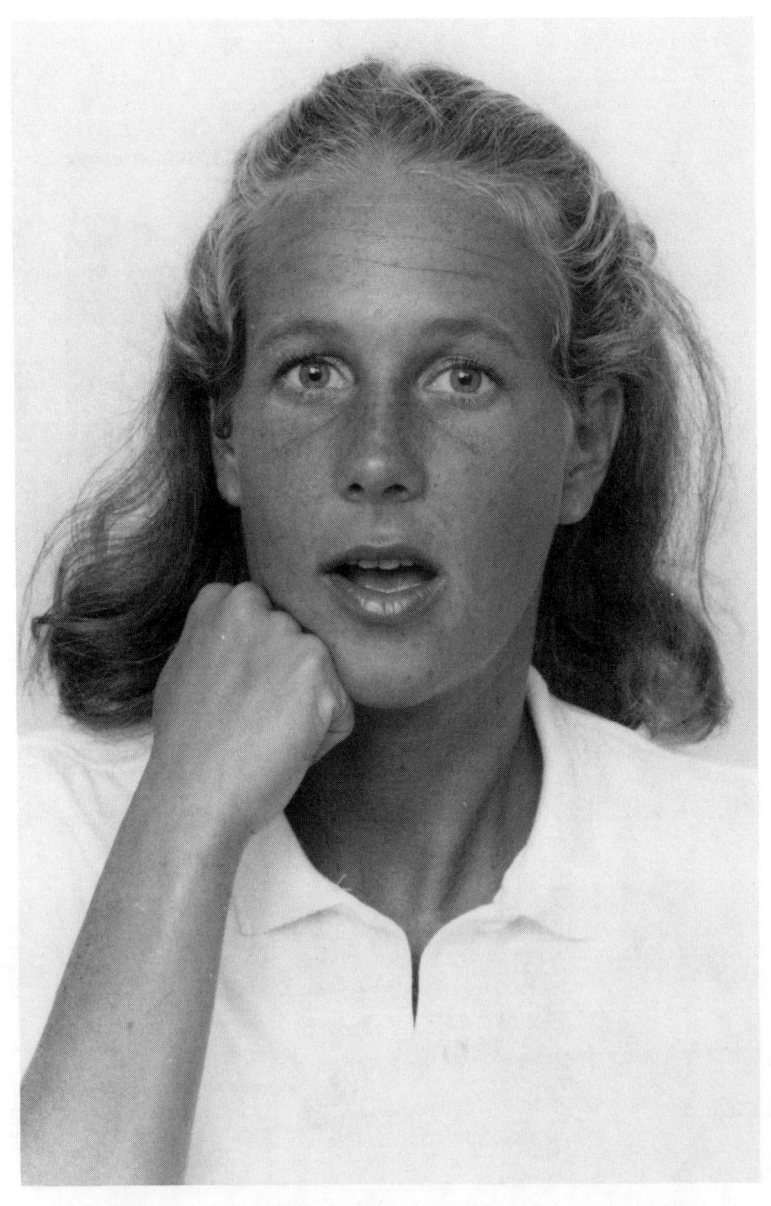

Figure 6-7. Active and passive exercises that reeducated and strengthen muscle groups.

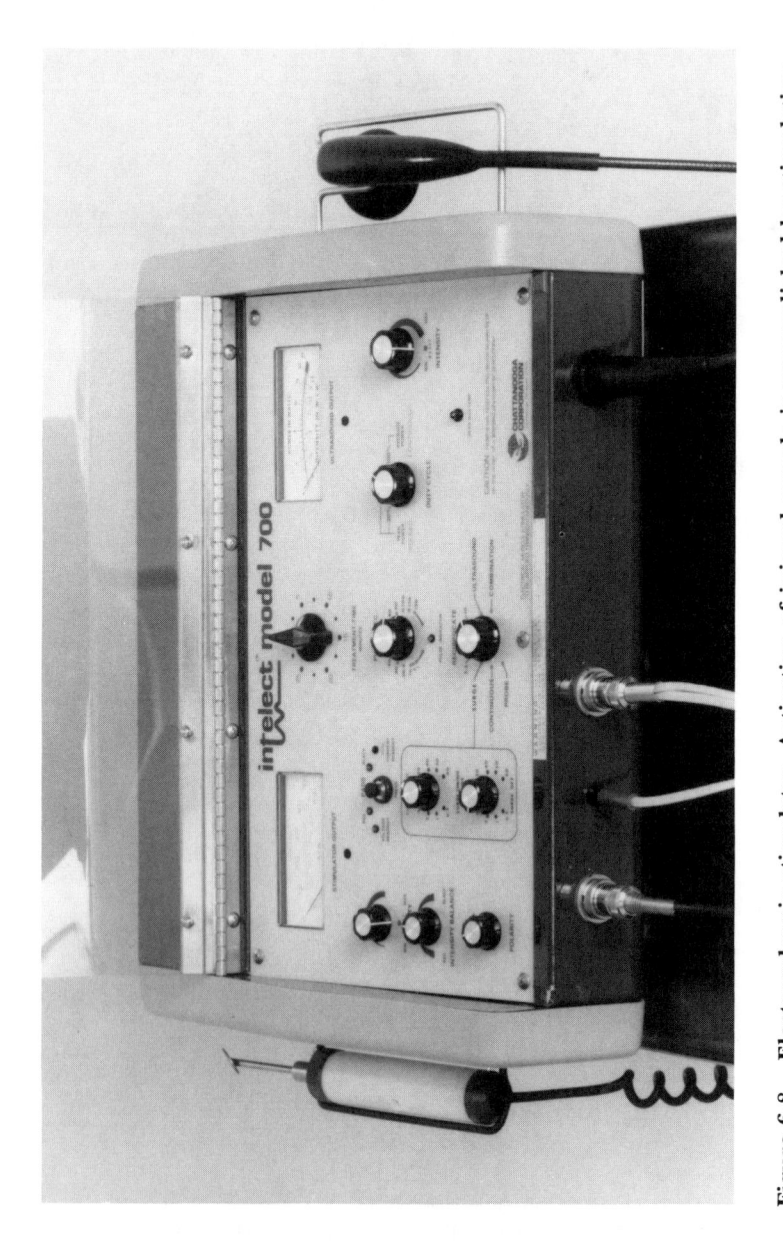

Figure 6-8. Electrogalvanic stimulator. Activation of injured muscle is accomplished by stimulating the nerve fiber or the muscle directly.

the muscle directly or its associated nerve. Both ultrasound therapy and electrical muscle stimulation are aimed at increasing circulation, reducing ischemia, and increasing elasticity of the muscle tissue.

Psychotherapy is not the initial treatment of choice for the patient with myofascial pain dysfunction syndrome; however, it may be of help in those patients who are nonresponsive to conservative treatment. Depression is often found to be the reason that many of these patients do not benefit from conventional treatment. Psychological counseling either on an individual basis or with group therapy may show improvement. Antidepressant medications, particularly the tricyclics, are very useful in reducing anxiety and altering sleep dysfunction. Amitriptyline in 50 to 150 mg dosages for 1 to 2 weeks at bedtime should be prescribed, especially if there is a concomitant sleep disturbance.

Patients who continue to be resistant to conservative treatment, or those who demonstrate a significant underlying psychological problem, may need referral to a psychiatrist for long-term psychotherapy. University-based pain centers specializing in the treatment of temporomandibular joint disorders and staffed by a group of multidisciplinary clinicians may be an alternative.

SUMMARY

Temporomandibular joint disorders can present a complex diagnostic problem. Due to the myriad of etiologies, differential diagnosis is difficult; however, this can be accomplished if a thorough approach is utilized. Distinguishing between complaints of pain (functional disorders) and complaints of dysfunction (structural disorders) is essential both for the clinician and the patient. Determination of the patient's primary etiology enables the clinician to formulate a proper differential diagnosis and treatment plan. A multidisciplinary and multidirectional team approach should be directed at the patient's principle problem; however, if both a functional and structural disorder are present, the functional disorder should be given priority.

An overview of temporomandibular joint disorders has been

presented in order to provide the clinician with the necessary information to render proper diagnosis and treatment.

References

1. McNeil C, Danzig W, Farrar WB, Gelb H, Lerman MC, Moffett BC, Pertes R, Solberg WK, Weinberg LA: Craniomandibular (TMJ) disorders—The state of the art. *J Prosthet Dent* 1980; 44:434.
2. Kreutziger KL, Mahan PE: Temporomandibular degenerative joint disease, Part I. *Oral Surg* 1975; 40:165.
3. Kreutziger KL, Mahan PE: Temporomandibular degenerative joint disease, Part II. *Oral Surg* 1975; 40:297.
4. Ogus H: Rheumatoid arthritis of the TMJ. *Br J Oral Surg* 1975; 12:275.
5. Poswillo D: Experimental investigation of the effects of intra-articular hydrocortisone with high condylectomy on the mandibular condyle. *Oral Surg* 1970; 30:161.
6. Irby, WB: *Current Advances in Oral Surgery* 1980; 3:291–299.
7. Irby WB: *Current Advances in Oral Surgery* 1980; 3:319–324.
8. Helms CA, Katzberg RW, Dolwick MF: *Internal Derangements of the Temporomandibular Joint.* Research and Education Foundation, 1983.
9. Katzberg RW, Dolwick MF, Bales DJ, Helms CA: Arthrography of the TMJ. *Am J of Radiology* 1979; 132:949–955.
10. Monson GS: Occlusion as applied to crown and bridge work. *J Natl Dent Assoc* 1920; 7:399–413.
11. Decker JC: Traumatic deafness as result of retrusion of condyles of mandible. *Ann Otol Rhinol Larynol* 1925; 34:519–527.
12. Costen JB: A syndrome of ear and sinus symptoms dependent upon disturbed function of the temporomandibular joint. *Ann Otol Rhinol Larynol* 1934; 43:1–15.
13. Sicher H: Temporomandibular articulation in mandibular overclosure. *JADA* 1948; 36:131–139.
14. Laskin DM: Etiology of the pain dysfunction syndrome. *JADA* 1969; 79:147–153.

15. Prentiss HJ: Preliminary report upon the temporomandibular articulation in the human. *Dent Cosmos* 1918; 60:505–512.
16. Sternbach R: *Pain Patients: Traits and Treatment.* New York, Academic, 1974.
17. Rugh JD: *A Behavioral Approach to Diagnosis and Treatment of Function Oral Disorders: Research and Clinical Applications.* Phoenix, Semantodontics, 1977.
18. Budzynski TH, Stoyva JM, Adler C: Feedback-induced muscle relaxation: Application to tension headache. *J Behav Ther Exp Psychiat* 1970; 1:205.
19. Curran JP: Skills training as an approach to the treatment of heterosexual–social anxiety: A review. *Psychol Bull* 1977; 84:140–157.
20. Tan SY: Cognitive and cognitive-behavioral methods for pain control: A selective review. *Pain* 1982; 12:201–228.
21. Ebershold MJ, Laws ER, Stonnington HH *et al:* Transcutaneous electrical stimulation for treatment of chronic pain: A preliminary report. *Surg Neurol* 1975; 4:96–99.
22. Loeser JD, Black RG, Christman A: Relief of pain by transcutaneous stimulation. *J Neurosurg* 1975; 42:308–314.
23. Melzack R: Prolonged relief of pain by brief intense transcutaneous somatic stimulation. *Pain* 1975; 1:357–373.
24. Melzack R, Wall PD: Pain mechanisms: A new theory. *Science* 1975; 150:971–979.
25. Sved A: Changing the occlusal level and a new method of retention. *Am J Orthod,* 1944; 30:527–535.
26. Hawley CA: A removable retainer. *Int J Orthod* 1919; 5:291–305.
27. Gelb H: *Clinical Management of Head, Neck and TMJ Pain and Dysfunction.* Philadelphia, W.B. Saunders, 1977.
28. Shore NA: Mandibular autorepositioning appliance. *JADA* 1967; 75:988–1011.
29. Rugh JD, Solberg WK: Electromyographic studies of bruxist behavior before and during treatment. *J Calif Dent Assoc* 1975; 3:56.

Chapter 7

IRRITABLE BOWEL SYNDROME

Michael E. McLeod, M.D.

INTRODUCTION

The functional or irritable bowel syndrome, although usually referring to colon disorders, can be viewed as including a spectrum of esophageal, gastric, and colonic derived symptoms. In this model a muscular digestive tube either has abnormal motility, or the sensations of normal motility are misperceived, resulting in the symptoms. More sophistication in the use of manometry, increasing knowledge of the enteric nervous system, and understanding of the link between the central nervous system and the intestinal tract with peptide hormones promise increasing understanding of normal and abnormal intestinal function in the future.[1] Despite gaps in our current knowledge, irritable bowel syndrome is an extremely important disorder for a number of reasons.

The first reason to devote an entire chapter to this topic is that this is a group of very common disorders. Epidemiological surveys suggest that up to 22 percent of the general population experience similar symptoms, even though a much smaller percentage actually seek medical attention.[2] Secondly, because the multiple symptoms, including nausea, vomiting, diarrhea, constipation, and abdominal pain, occur in the setting of normal laboratory and X-ray studies, there is a great deal of misunderstanding by both patient and physician as to the nature of the problem. Patients find it hard to understand how the bloating, tender palpable masses (loops of distended bowel) and diarrhea can occur, and everything be "normal." Physicians, in addition, frequently tell patients to "learn to live with it," without attempting to explain the mechanism of the symptoms or to educate the patient on how to alter the pattern of symptoms. Finally, the combination of symptoms, in particular the abdominal pain reported by the patients, frequently leads to unnecessary medical and surgical therapy. In many instances, surgery is carried out for gallstones, hiatus hernia, diverticular disease, hysterectomy, or removal of adhesions when, in fact, the symptoms reported by the patient are unrelated to the findings on X ray or at surgery.

Three distinctions are of major importance in understanding the irritable bowel syndrome: 1) functional versus organic; 2) disease versus illness; and 3) psychological stress. "Organic" has been used in the past to denote situations with anatomical and histological abnormalities, whereas "functional" implies absence of these abnormalities. Because structural abnormalities are lacking in functional diagnoses they are often equated with the psychogenic, neurotic, or even imaginary.

The era of electron microscopy and molecular biology has allowed us to focus on disease at levels beyond the cellular. For example, lactase deficiency and Acute Intermittent Porphyria are molecular diseases, with specific treatment now available, that previously would have been identified as "functional." In exploring patients' symptoms, we must ask at what level are we to look for their disease, i.e., gross or microscopic anatomy, molecular abnormalities, abnormal motility, or other undefined level. In addition, the duration of the abnormality and method of measurement are important. Ulcers last for weeks, erosions may last for days, and gastritis induced by alcohol may last for hours. Spasm in the esophagus may be present for seconds to minutes. Hence, depending on whether we use X ray, endoscopic exam, or motility measurements may determine whether or not we define an abnormality. If we do define an abnormality, we must attempt to see if it correlates with the patient's symptoms.

The second distinction is disease versus illness.[3] Disease is a biological event with anatomical, physiological, and biochemical changes in the person. These may or may not cause an illness, i.e., a change in the patient in terms of symptoms or performance level. Asymptomatic coronary disease, silent peptic ulcer, G6-PD deficiency, and silent gallstones represent molecular and anatomical diseases that can be present without the patient experiencing symptoms. Illness, on the other hand, is the experience of the patient in terms of 1) pain or discomfort; 2) alterations in performance levels, such as weakness, fatigability, or anorexia, and 3) specific abnormality in body functions such as breathing, swallowing, defecation, etc. Again, it must be emphasized that the patient's illness may not correlate with the disease as we define it in terms of our X-ray, endoscopic, laboratory or molecular abnormalities. The patient who is bloating and belching and complaining of upper abdominal pressure after each meal will not be helped by cholecystectomy except through its potential placebo effect.

Finally, how can the concept of psychological stress be integrated into this model? Psychological stress can be defined as any process within the person or the environment that creates a demand, the resolution of which will demand mental work. Usually this involves loss or threat of loss, injury or threat of injury, or frustration of an inner drive or need. It is important to emphasize that stress occurs in all individuals. Some stress is important in terms of normal growth and change as human beings. However, if stress accumulates and exceeds a certain threshold, certain physiological changes may occur in many organ systems, ranging from elevations in blood pressure to bronchospasm to changes in intestinal motility. The pattern of organ response may in large part be genetically determined. Many patients will report only the somatic symptoms and have no associated emotional component, while other patients will experience the feelings of rage, fear, or sadness along with the physiological event described above. There are some universal stressors, such as major losses, including death of a spouse or loved one, loss of a job, or loss of an organ, such as breast or colon. Major surgery or life-threatening accidents also represent universal stresses.

However, there are certain stresses that are conditioned or learned in response to each patient's unique past history. A roller coaster ride may be exciting to some individuals, but represent a major threat to others. Type "A" personalities are stressed by their self-imposed time pressures, which are internally generated. There are some data suggesting that despite similar or different stressful stimuli, the responsive organ system may be unique to the individual, perhaps genetically determined, as in certain familial peptic ulcer syndromes, or in patients with hyperactive airways, seen in the asthmatic population.[4] Additionally, there are situations in which there is a reward maintenance system with increasing family attention, avoidance of responsibilities, i.e., the "sick role," leading to secondary gain in the situation and perpetuation of the symptom complex.

Functional bowel syndrome is a heterogeneous group of disorders with symptoms originating from three portions of the gastrointestinal tract: esophageal, with the patient presenting with intermittent chest pain and dysphagia; gastric, in which the patient presents with nausea, early satiety, bloating, and pain; colonic, in which the patient's complaints relate to pain, bloating, and change in bowel pattern. The general conceptual model frequently used to explain these disorders is that of a hollow muscular tube, capable of regular, rhythmic, sequential, and propulsive contractions, which in certain locations and under certain conditions may develop simultaneous contraction waves with changes in intensity, amplitude, and duration of contraction, producing retrograde flow and distention and, at times, partial obstruction. As a result, normal function is interrupted and the symptoms result.

ESOPHAGEAL MOTILITY DISORDERS

Esophageal motility disorders are more easily defined because of easier access and less complexity than the gastric and colon disorders. There are primary muscle disorders such as achalasia and diffuse esophageal spasm with well-defined manometric criteria. There are also secondary muscular disorders such as the hyperdynamic or "nutcracker" esophagus in which the abnormal motility occurs in several situations and appears to be secondary to other factors. In this group, the abnormal motility may be correlated with signs and symptoms of increasing emotional and psychological stress and many of these patients fit specific psychiatric diagnoses as defined by *Diagnostic and Statistical Manual of Mental Disorders,* Third Edition, published by the American Psychiatric Association in 1980. In addition, mucosal and inflammatory changes such as reflux esophagitis may contribute to this abnormal motility pattern. The pain is typically described as squeezing, pressing, and substernal in location, frequently radiating to the back and neck. These patients may experience difficulty with swallowing, including solids and liquids; a food bolus will frequently stop abruptly, followed in several minutes by relief. The pain and dysphagia may occur separately or simultaneously. In this group of patients, endoscopic examination is important to exclude inflammatory changes, and motility studies are needed to determine the presence or absence of primary muscle disorders, i.e., achalasia and diffuse esophageal spasm. Since stress and associated psychological factors are often felt to be important, other changes in performance levels should be looked for including changes in energy level, early morning fatigue, altered sleep pattern, recurrent headaches, or altered moods. Stable weight, hemoglobin, normal albumin and Westergren sedimentation rate also help support this diagnosis.

Because esophageal motility disorders may produce substernal pressure and pain mimicking cardiac disease, this is a common clinical problem for cardiologists. Wells and Lustman reported 50 patients with negative coronary angiograms and atypical chest pain.[5] Esophageal motility studies demonstrated that 25 of 50 had abnormal studies compatible with "nutcracker" or hyperdynamic esophagus. The 25 patients underwent psychological testing using stringent criteria outlined in *DSM*-III and 85 percent had a positive diagnosis, including 13 with depression, five with somatization disorder, nine with generalized, anxiety and seven with phobia. A control population had only 31 percent positive with *DSM*-III diagnosis. This study showed an increased association of atypical chest pain, negative angiograms, and abnormal esophageal motility, with an increased prevalence of psychiatric illness. The direct relationship of the pain to the motility pattern was not established in this study. In other studies, however, similar patients infused with Tensilon or ergonovine have had their chest pain reproduced with simultaneous esophageal spasm noted on manometry.

Gastric Disorders

Gastric disorders include patients with 1) nausea, vomiting, early satiety in the setting of normal endoscopy; 2) aerophagia with bloating and abdominal distention frequently relieved by belching; 3) pain diffusely located, migrating to different quadrants of the abdomen vaguely described with multiple adjectives such as burning, aching, pressure, stabbing, etc. The symptoms vary in relationship to time of day and meals and tend to occur several days per week, rarely remitting more than a week. Symptoms are rarely nocturnal except in patients with depression where there may be early morning awakening between 3 and 5 a.m. In contrast, peptic ulcer disease tends to wake patients between midnight and 2 a.m., generally manifests daily pain, and has a clear relation to meals, with food either relieving or aggravating the pain. When these multiple gastric symptoms have been present intermittently for years with previous negative X rays and endoscopy, the diagnosis is not difficult. However, the onset of new symptoms of this type in a patient over fifty years of age in the absence of previous psychophysiologic disorders should prompt careful examination to exclude other diseases such as gastric ulcer and gastric malignancy.

Gastric motility measurements are still at a level of research interest and do not provide clinical help in managing these types of patients.

Colonic Disorders

The third and final group is the irritable colon syndrome or spastic colon, the most common of the three groups. Estimates suggest that up to 50 percent of consults to gastroenterologists are referred for this disorder.[2] Unfortunately, there is no motility pattern that has been documented to be specific for this disorder. However, clinical criteria have been proposed by Manning et al.[6] and include:

1) abdominal pain present in any or all four quadrants including lower chest and subscapular region. The lower abdominal area is the most common site, with pain lasting from 5 to 30 minutes. The pain tends to be migratory and frequently is associated with abdominal distention and bloating and at times with palpable loops of bowel. The pain is often relieved by bowel movement or passage of flatus and frequently occurs with loose bowel movements, obstipation, or frequent defecation with normal bowel consistency. The various pain types including the subscapular and lower chest pains have been reproduced in over 50 percent of one group of patients using colonoscopy and distensible balloon.

2) Altered bowel pattern is an almost universal complaint. Constipation with tapered bowel movements which fluctuate from normal caliber to narrow stool caliber indicating a variable degree of obstruction rather than the fixed obstruction of carcinoma is a frequent complaint. The pattern of alternating diarrhea and constipation is also common.

3) Abdominal bloating and distention are frequent symptoms. These often become worse as the day progresses and may or may not be relieved with passage of gas. Actual measurements of methane, hydrogen, and nitrogen indicate that the majority of patients with functional colon syndrome do not pass excessive gas, but appear to handle it differently in terms of their motility pattern.[7] Levitt has shown that by perfusion of argon gas into the bowel of patients with irritable bowel syndrome they report many more symptoms than the control population with the same volume of infused gas.

4) Increased passage of mucus is often noted.

5) The sensation of incomplete rectal emptying is also frequently reported. Proctalgia fugax or intense pain within the rectum lasting minutes and occurring spontaneously is much less frequent.

The more these symptoms are reported to the exclusion of factors listed below will increase the sensitivity and specificity of the diagnosis of functional colon syndrome. The important exclusions include 1) significant weight loss, 2) blood loss except that identified as from the anal canal, 3) lactose intolerance, 4) abnormal hemoglobin, albumin, and Westergren sedimentation rate, 5) abnormal proctoscopy and barium enema. The latter examinations are a minimum for patients over forty and in younger patients with symptoms of recent onset and intractable clinical illness. The proctoscopy is directed at excluding inflammatory changes and examining the stool microscopically for white cells and parasites.

6) A pelvic examination should be carried out to exclude ovarian malignancy involving the colon, and to rule out subacute inflammatory disease of the pelvic organs. The presence of weight loss, progressive pattern of symptoms, occurrence in older age group, and brief duration of symptoms with no previous psychophysiologic disorder should alert one to the possibility of another process. The symptoms of the irritable bowel patient can be identical to those of the patient who has partial obstructing rectosigmoid carcinoma except for the shorter duration of symptoms, associated blood, abnormal proctoscopic exam, etc. In addition, patients with the functional colon syndrome are obviously not immune to developing other gastrointestinal diseases and should be periodically reevaluated. Following these patients serially will be important to provide support and identify new symptoms or variations of old symptoms that could suggest a new problem.

In addition, the presence of an organic process should not exclude a component of functional bowel. Some patients with ulcerative proctitis will experience bloating and alternating diarrhea, and constipation as part of their functional irritable bowel syndrome, and this will make it difficult at times to separate which process is most active. Similarly, secondary spasm and pain in reflux esophagitis may be related more to associated depression and anxiety than the actual peptic inflammation. The persistence of symptoms during therapy in this situation may be related more to the treatment being directed only at the peptic component. Anxiety and depression are great amplifiers of symptoms as well as producers of symptoms.

Once alternative diseases have been excluded, education is the first step in treatment. The patient must have a clear understanding of the symptoms and the mechanism of their production. Pain, diarrhea, and dysphagia are not imaginary symptoms. The patient's anxiety regarding these symptoms and what they imply, i.e., fear of cancer, surgery, or starvation is frequently adding to their current life stresses.[8] The patient can frequently palpate distended bowel loops, will observe his abdomen to swell, and may experience severe pain. If patients are taught that these alterations can occur as a result of focal changes in bowel motility this begins to provide some explanation for their problem and will help relieve their anxiety. Physician awareness of the importance of the placebo effect is also important. Multiple studies have shown that approximately 30 to 35 percent of patients will improve with placebo despite the nature of their illness.[9] Medical and surgical procedures carried out in patients with irritable bowel syndrome frequently result in transient improvement, only to have the patient return weeks to months later with relapse of their symptoms, resulting in frustration for the patient and the physician. Surgery, in particular, has a powerful placebo effect and it is not uncommon for these patients to be relieved of symptoms for 3 to 6 months after surgery for adhesions, hernia repair, cholecystectomy, etc., when the anatomical correction had nothing to do with the patient's original symptoms. It must be emphasized that a symptomatic improvement in response to a specific therapy does not confirm a specific pathophysiologic illness. It is apparent from studies carried out by Alpers in functional colon disorders[10] and Wells and Lustman in esophageal disorders[5] that 72 to 83 percent of these patients will have specific psychiatric diagnoses, compared to 18 to 31 percent of controls. Many patients may be involved in anxiety-producing situations that are limited in duration, and the symptoms may resolve as the anxiety subsides. It should be emphasized that any of the functional bowel syndromes, whether they are esophageal, gastric, or colonic, may occur in any of a variety of psychiatric diagnoses, ranging from situational anxiety, depression, somatization disorder, or phobic disorders. Each of these labels will carry a different prognosis and require different treatment, although the bowel symptoms may be identical. Environmental stressors should always be looked for as precipitating factors. According to Alpers, depression appears to be one of the diagnoses most commonly missed by internists, an important diagnosis because it may be amenable to tricyclic therapy.[10] Patients must be educated as to the potential role of stress in their illness and be helped in assuming responsibility for changing that part of their life. This might include behavioral tasks like making up list of stress-producing situations and identifying which situation may be changeable. Regular exercise will also be effective in reducing general stress, and relaxation therapy including meditation and biofeedback is often helpful. The patient will need to understand that the disorder will fluctuate depending on ability to control the stress in his life. The evaluation of the role of stress will be difficult at times and will depend on the type, intensity, duration of the stress, and the presence or absence of a support system in the environment. Psychotherapy will be appropriate for those motivated to pursue their stressors more thoroughly.

Treatment of the esophageal disorders should be directed at the mucosal inflammatory process and the specific environmental stresses as noted above. Specific relaxation of the muscle can be carried out using nitrites and calcium channel blockers. However, these agents are more effective in the primary muscle disorders. Anticholinergics and mild sedatives can be used in both esophageal and gastric disorders, but tend to produce disagreeable side effects and have never been shown in any control studies to be more effective than a placebo. The colon disorder group can be helped by providing more bulk, including bran, Metamucil, or high fiber diets that can help stabilize the bowel pattern and avoid either obstipation or diarrhea.[11] We must understand that we are treating symptoms with these various programs and our goal should be to alleviate or reduce the causal factors where they are identifiable. In all functional gastrointestinal disorders the symptomatic treatment should not supercede the identification and treatment of stress, the psychological component.

REFERENCES

1. Stranghellini JR, Malagelada JR, Go VLW, Kao PC: Stress-induced gastroduodenal motor disturbance in humans: Possible humoral mechanisms. *Gastroenterology* 1983;85:85.

2. Sandler RS et al: Symptom complaints and health care seeking behavior in subjects with bowel dysfunction. *Gastroenterology* 1984;87:314.
3. Barondess J: Disease and illness—A crucial distinction. *Amer J Med* 1979;66:375.
4. Engel G: The need for a new medical model: A challenge for biomedicine. *Science* 1977;196 (4286):129–135.
5. Clouse RE, Lustman PJ: Psychiatric illness and contraction abnormalities of the esophagus. *N Eng J Med* 1983;309:1337.
6. Manning AP et al: Towards positive diagnosis of the irritable bowel syndrome. *Br Med J* 1978;2:658.
7. Volume and composition of human intestinal gas determined by means of an intestinal washout technique. *N Eng J Med* 1971;284:1394.
8. Wiggins K: How fear affects medical symptoms. *Physician and Patient*, April 1983, p.10.
9. Kirsner J: Irritable bowel syndrome: Clinical review and ethical considerations. *Arch Int Med* 1981;141:635.
10. Alpers D: Functional gastrointestinal disorders. *Hosp Prac*, April 1983, p. 139.
11. Drossman D, Powell D, Sessions JT: Irritable bowel syndrome: Clinical gastroenterology conference. *Gastroenterology* 1977;73:811.

Chapter 8

PERINEAL PAIN

Prostatodynia or Prostatitis?

Culley C. Carson III, M.D.

INTRODUCTION

Perineal pain symptoms are similar in prostatitis and non-prostatitis-type syndromes. Those symptoms include burning on urination or dysuria, urgency and frequency of urination, as well as low back pain, perineal pain and aching, scrotalgia, and lower abdominal pain. Frequently patients have postejaculatory pain; that is, pain or burning in the pelvis after ejaculation. Postejaculatory pain is a hallmark of prostatitis-associated symptoms. Patients who do not have stress-related prostatic symptoms, but rather bacterial prostatitis, may also have symptoms of chills and fever, hematuria, urinary retention, and epididymitis. We take up each of these symptoms and signs, and discuss them in more detail.

Prostatodynia concerns primarily the symptoms associated with perineal pain in the male. How do we make the diagnosis of stress-related perineal pain in contradistinction to specific diseases that cause the same kinds of symptoms? What are some of the possible causes of the nonprostatitis-type perineal pain? What are the treatments?

Definitions

Before 1978, the prostatitis-type syndromes were classified as acute prostatitis, chronic prostatitis, and prostatosis. Acute prostatitis is a urologic emergency, and may result in gram-negative sepsis. Chronic prostatitis included bacterial and nonbacterial forms of prostatitis. The word prostatosis means "process of the prostate" and, because of the somewhat nonsensical nature of that term, the prostatitis-type syndromes were reclassified in 1978.[1] The classification that we presently use to discuss the different kinds of prostatic syndromes includes acute bacterial prostatitis, chronic bacterial prostatitis, nonbacterial prostatitis, and prostatodynia. In this schema, acute bacterial prostatitis and chronic bacterial prostatitis also involve specific bacteria causing infection in the prostate. Nonbacterial prostatitis is a similar condition in which infective agents in the prostate are not typical bacterial pathogens. Finally, for this discussion, "prostatosis" is replaced by the word "prostatodynia," which means "pain in the prostate."

Etiological Agents

Symptoms of bacterial prostatitis occur in a bimodal curve, occuring in the twenty- to forty-year age group, and then again from fifty-five to seventy. It is important to note that bacterial prostatitis begins to decline after about age sixty-nine, and if a patient in his early seventies presents with new symptoms of perineal pain and no symptoms of prostatitis in the past, carcinoma of the prostate must be considered. Some urologists feel that a patient over seventy who has new prostatitis has prostatic cancer, until proven otherwise. In this group of patients, attributing symptoms of prostatitis to stress or even to bacterial infections must only be done by exclusion of carcinoma.

Bacterial prostatitis can be caused by gram-negative infections, most commonly *E. coli*, or by gram-positive organisms, most commonly *Staphylococcus aureus* or other staphylococci.[2,3,4] Prostatodynia and nonbacterial prostatitis are not caused by bacterial organisms. Anaerobic bacteria, trichomonas and *Herpes simplex* virus have been eliminated as causes of nonbacterial prostatitis or prostatodynia. *Ureaplasma urealyticum* and chlamydia, however, continue to be somewhat controversial. If one cultures the posterior urethra of a patient with prostatic symptoms, one will most likely find either *U. urealyticum* or chlamydia in the culture; however, one is also likely to find those same organisms in the culture of asymptomatic patients.[5,6] Whether or not these agents are the cause of symptoms remains controversial. An allergic or immunologic cause has also been suggested and, in fact, some patients' symptoms will respond to a food elimination diet. If they do respond to these diets, they will usually respond to elimination of chocolate, caffeine, alcohol, or tomato products. This group, however, is quite small, and these patients almost always have a strong allergic history, and may have large quantities of eosinophils in their prostatic fluid.

Chemical prostatitis is a frequent cause of prostatodynia in the older man. These symptoms occur primarily as a result of marginal or mild obstructive symptoms caused by benign prostatic hypertrophy, and may respond to surgical relief of obstruction.

CLINICAL AND LABORATORY EVALUATION

In order to differentiate these prostatic problems, one must begin by a proper examination of the prostate and a prostatic massage. The prostates in all of these patients are tender to palpation. The tenderness is usually most marked at the base of the prostate. The best way to rule out infectious causes is to perform a prostatic massage, beginning at the lateral border of the prostate and massaging medially all along each prostatic lobe to the midline, and finally stripping the urethra in the midline to completely examine the prostate and to obtain prostatic fluid for microscopic evaluation and culture.

Once a prostatic massage has been performed, the next goal is to eliminate infection as the cause of the perineal pain. The differential culture method described by Meares and Stamey is the best method to culture prostatic fluid.[7] The patient arrives for evaluation with a full bladder, and he voids the first 10 ml of urine, which is sent to the laboratory as the VB1 culture (voided bladder number one), and represents the urethral washings. The patient voids another 100 to 200 ml volume of urine and collects a midstream specimen, which is labelled VB2 and represents s the midstream or the bladder urine culture. Voiding is stopped and a prostatic massage is performed as described. After massage some EPS (expressed prostatic secretions) are collected, if available. Usually the EPS volume is not large and EPS cannot always be cultured. Some of these secretions, however, can be placed on a glass slide for microscopic evaluation. The patient then gives his next 10 ml of voided urine after the prostatic massage. This VB3 (voided bladder number three) specimen will wash the posterior urethra, and will bring with it some prostatic fluid which can then be cultured to determine if bacterial prostatitis is present. Usually the VB2 is clear, but the VB3 specimen will have a large number of bacteria if there is a chronic bacterial prostatitis. Likewise, the expressed prostatic secretions, if enough was collected, will give a positive culture. If there are some bacteria in the bladder, the VB3 colony count must be at least one log higher than the VB2 count to be significant.[8]

Microscopic examination of the EPS can make an immediate diagnosis in the office. The EPS specimen will reveal several findings in a patient with a prostatic infection. The number of white blood cells or "pus cells" present in the specimen and lipid laden macrophages or oval fat bodies are important while so-called lecithin granules probably are not of great importance.[9] As many as 12 white blood cells per high power field are within the norm for prostatic fluid. More than 12 cells will indicate the probability of bacterial infectious prostatitis. In bacterial prostatitis, an increase in white blood cells, an increase in oval fat bodies, and a decrease in lecithin granules are usually present in prostatic secretions. The typical expressed prostatic secretion in a patient with bacterial prostatitis has a large number of white blood cells containing inclusion bodies. Phase contrast microscopy shows these double refractile oval fat bodies very clearly. . In nonbacterial prostatitis, that is, prostatitis caused by some other infectious agent but with negative standard cultures, an increase in white blood cells also occurs. Oval fat bodies and changes in the lecithin granules are usually present in this group of patients as well.

Patients with prostatodynia have pure stress-related symptoms of perineal pain and prostatic inflammation and will have few white blood cells in their prostatic fluid. There is no increase in oval fat bodies and lecithin granules are variable. Selective cultures of prostatic fluid have no growth. Nilsson and coworkers performed MMPI's on a group of patients who had long-term prostatodynia which was prostatic fluid culture negative and microscopic secretion negative and found significant elevations in the psychosis and paranoia scales.[10] Also identified were defects in sexual identification, a finding that has not been previously reported in association with prostatodynia.

There is a segment of patients with prostatodynia who present somewhat atypically and have symptoms of urinary obstruction. The symptoms are similar to benign prostatic hypertrophy, but also include perineal and postejaculatory pain. Most commonly these patients have hesitancy on urination, decreased urinary stream, double voiding, nocturia, and frequency. They rarely have complete urinary retention. Cystometrograms of these patients may show spasm of the external urinary sphincter, decreased urine flow rate, incomplete funnelling of the bladder neck during voiding and urethral narrowing at the external sphincter. These findings suggest a sympathetic nerve function abnormality causing incomplete relaxation of the urethral musculature.[11] These patients can be treated with phenoxybenzamine 10 mg at bedtime. Usually a 21- to 30-day course of phenoxybenzamine in these patients will improve obstructive symptoms, and frequently will eliminate perineal pain. However, in patients with prostatodynia without obstructive symptoms, this regimen is rarely successful.

In summary, the key point in differentiation of perineal pain caused by infection or psychophysiologic syndrome is the expressed prostatic secretions. Office examination of these secretions is a simple matter, and can be performed easily after prostatic examination. The patients with bacterial and nonbacterial prostatitis will have markedly elevated prostatic fluid white blood cell counts, while those with prostatodynia will be normal. The oval fat bodies will be elevated in infectious types of prostatitis, and the cultures will be positive only with bacterial prostatitis.

TREATMENT

How does one best treat patients with prostatodynia and perineal pain? This is a subject of controversy as no good series of patients has been reported with significant success in eliminating the symptoms of prostatodynia. If a patient has increased white blood cells on expressed prostatic secretions with a negative culture, we generally treat with tetracycline or erythromycin, since their perineal pain may be caused by *Ureaplasma urealyticum* or chlamydia. This course of medication must be maintained for a period of 4 to 6 weeks, with examination of their prostatic secretions prior to discontinuing medication. Repeated prostatic massage is no longer appropriate treatment of these patients; however, most patients do respond well to frequent ejaculations, since frequent ejaculation is more effective than prostatic massage in expressing prostatic fluid. Antihistamines are helpful only in that group of patients who have large numbers of eosinophils in their prostatic fluid. Antihistamines themselves, especially those in many of the over-the-counter cold remedies associated with decongestants, may add to the external sphincter spasm in those patients who have obstructive symptoms. Antihistamines are thus contraindicated in those patients who have obstructive symptoms and associated perineal pain.

Transurethral prostatectomy is likewise contraindicated in patients with prostatodynia. It has been said that if one operates for pain, that is what one will find. In fact, that is true with transurethral prostatectomy for perineal pain; if one operates on perineal pain, the patient frequently will be back with more pain postoperatively. Hot sitz baths are helpful, and can be therapeutic in some cases. We have successfully used biofeedback techniques on occasion, but this is best reserved for patients who have specific, definable external sphincter spasm.[12]

The treatment of most of these patients is supportive. Evaluation of anxiety and stress relationships is important and these factors should be modified when possible. The patient should be aware that recurrences may occur during periods of stress. Symptomatic support includes frequent ejaculations, hot sitz baths, mild analgesics or nonsteroidal anti-inflammatory agents, and avoidance of caffeine and alcohol.

References

1. Drach GW, Fair WR, Meares EM, Stamey TA: Classification of benign diseases associated with prostatic pain: Prostatitis or prostatodynia (letter). *J Urol* 1978; 120:266.
2. Meares EM: Bacterial prostatitis vs "prostatosis": A clinical and bacteriological study. *JAMA* 1973; 224:1372.
3. Carson CC, McGraw VD, Zwadyk P: Bacterial prostatitis caused by Staphylococcus saprophyticus. *Urology* 1982; 6:165.
4. Drach GW: Problems in diagnosis of bacterial prostatitis: Gram negative, gram positive and mixed infections. *J Urol* 1974; 111:630.
5. Weidner W *et al:* Qualitative culture of Ureaplasma urealiticum in patients with chronic prostatitis or prostatosis. *J Urol* 1980; 124:622.
6. Berger RE *et al:* Chlamydia trachomatis as a cause of acute idiopathic epididymitis. *NEJM* 1978; 298:301.
7. Meares EM, Stamey TA: Bacteriologic localization patterns in bacterial prostatitis and urethritis. *Invest Urol* 1968; 5:492.
8. Carson CC: Urinary tract infection. In Resnick MI, Older RA (Eds), *Diagnosis of Genitourinary Disease.* New York, Thieme-Stratton, 1982.
9. Anderson RU, Weller C: Prostatic secretion leukocyte studies in non-bacterial prostatitis (prostatosis). *J Urol* 1979; 121:292.
10. Nilsson IK, Colleen S, Mardh PA: Relationship between psychological and laboratory findings in patients with symptoms of non-acute prostatitis. In Danielson D, Juhlin L, Mardh PA (Eds), *Genital Infections and Their Complications.* Stockholm, Almquist and Wiksell International, 1975.
11. Barbalias GA, Meares EM, Sant GR: Prostatodynia: Clinical and urodynamic characteristics. *J Urol* 1983; 130:275.
12. Segura JW, Opitz, JL, Greene LF: Prostatosis, prostatitis or pelvic floor tension myalgia? *J Urol* 1979; 122:168.

Chapter 9

THE CHRONIC PAIN PATIENT

Behavioral Treatment Strategies

John S. Jordan, Ph.D.
Francis J. Keefe, Ph.D.

Tom Davis is a forty-two-year-old construction worker who has been out of work 9 months because of pain in his back and legs. Tom says he is unable to do anything around the house because the pain is so severe. He finds it difficult to sleep. His formerly robust appetite is gone, and he spends almost all of his day on the couch reclining. Tom's wife is upset and doesn't know what do. She finds that she has had to take over most of the responsibilities around the house and even has to do simple things for her husband like tying his shoes because he is unable to bend down. She says that Tom has become a hermit, won't tell her what is on his mind, and even refuses to return telephone calls to friends and other family. Tom has seen numerous doctors, and all agree that he shouldn't have another back surgery. While many different medications have been tried, none seem to work, and Tom finds he needs to take more and more to get any pain relief at all.

Tom Davis is like millions of other chronic pain patients. His life has become dominated by pain to the extent that he focuses on little else. Managing patients like Tom is extremely frustrating and difficult. Most of these patients have exhausted surgical treatment alternatives and fail to respond to pharmacologic approaches. As pain persists, significant behavioral and psychological problems develop that make their treatment even more difficult.

Until recently, there have been relatively few options for management of the patient with intractable pain. Specialized pain clinics and pain management programs have been developed and refined since the mid-1970s.[1] They are based upon a single assumption: Chronic pain is a complex problem that requires a comprehensive team-oriented approach directed not only at the somatic component of pain but also behavioral and psychological reactions to pain. Several research reviews indicate that specialized inpatient programs help many patients who have failed to respond to previous treatment efforts.[2,3]

In this chapter, we focus on one component of a multidisciplinary approach to chronic pain: behavioral intervention strategies. This chapter is divided into two sections. The first section presents a brief overview of the basic concepts underlying behavioral treatment strategies. In the second section, we review in detail a behavioral treatment process from initial evaluation through treatment and follow-up.

Basic Concepts

Conditioning and Learning

According to the behavioral perspective, the development and persistence of chronic pain can be influenced greatly by learning and social factors. Fundamental to this perspective is the principle of reinforcement. Simplistically stated, behaviors that decrease/avoid punishment or increase pleasure will be repeated under similar future circumstances.

Pain can be a potent punishment and hence a powerful factor in learning. For most people, this has positive and adaptive consequences. Every pain episode is not a completely new, trial-and-error learning experience. Instead, people readily repeat those responses that bring them pain relief (e.g., medication, bed rest). They also learn to avoid those actions that seem to result in increased pain (e.g., lifting, reaching, bending) and become increasingly adept at detecting nociceptive cues. Such cues serve as warning signals that often give rise to what we call "pain behaviors" (e.g., moaning, limping, rubbing, bracing, grimacing). Initially some of these "pain behaviors" may actually function to avoid or reduce pain. However, because pain behaviors are observable, they also tend to elicit sympathetic and nurturant (i.e., rewarding) responses from significant others. While substantial behavioral changes often accompany acute pain, such changes are usually temporary. After a brief recovery period, most acute pain patients return to relatively normal daily functioning.

Other individuals, however, do not regain a functional lifestyle. These chronic pain patients consistently tell us that their activity patterns are unmoderated, unstable, and unpredictable; they go between extremes of inactivity and overdoing. As chronic pain lingers or worsens, their periods of inactivity get longer and longer. Eventually many such patients report being in bed all but a few hours per day. The same behaviors that may have served adaptively during acute pain develop a "life of their own," an existence no longer tied directly to nociception. These individuals have become trapped in a pain cycle, the basic elements of which are displayed in the lower right portion of Figure 9-1.

The Pain Cycle

When they "finally feel good enough to be active," chronic pain patients are usually *overactive,* attempting "get it all in while they can." As a result of "overdoing," pain is significantly intensified. Extreme pain results in excessive "pain behaviors" (e.g., rubbing, moaning, and grimacing) and attempts intended to reduce the pain (e.g., taking narcotic medications, getting prolonged rest, staying out of work). These actions are often extremely reinforcing. Unfortunately, the patient learns that such rewards are contingent on the presence of pain (i.e., no pain—no rewards). Also, because observable pain behaviors often elicit unusually nurturant and supportive responses from others, the pain behaviors themselves are rewarded. Often unintentionally, pain behaviors then are repeated irrespective of nociception to obtain the desired reinforcers.

Figure 9-1.

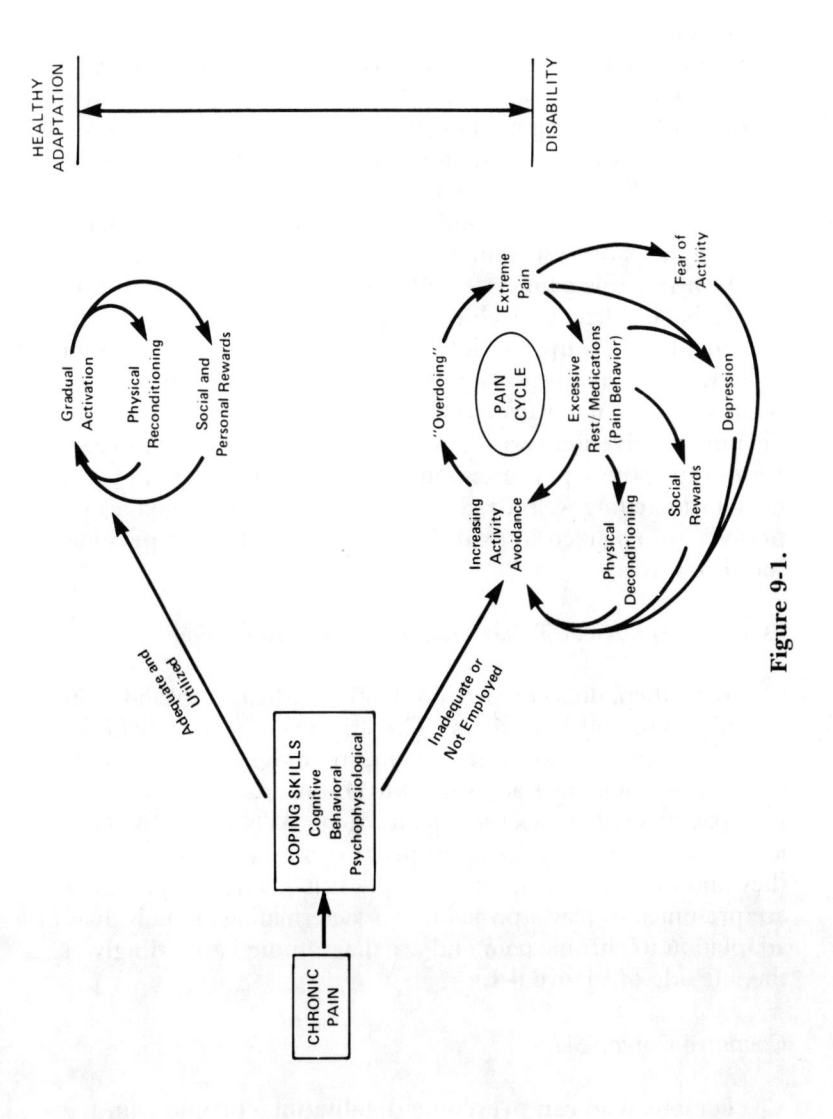

In this scenario, perceived pain and pain behaviors are rewarded and activity is punished. Activity therefore becomes increasingly avoided—even feared. "Recovery periods" between episodes of overdoing get longer and longer. Over time, reductions in activity level also diminish physical stamina, making future activity that much more difficult and/or painful. The pain cycle—decreasing activity and increasing pain behaviors, medication usage, and rest—builds on itself unless somehow broken.

Contrast this pain cycle with the pattern of activity and rewards that can lead to healthy, adaptive functioning. This is diagrammed in this upper right portion of Figure 1. Activity is moderated so as not to significantly exacerbate pain. Instead, regular, modulated activity results in physical reconditioning and permits involvement with rewarding and meaningful events. Significant others pay attention to (and reward) these approximations to getting well. Gradually, increasingly prolonged activity periods are engaged in (with increasing potential for personal/social reward).

Psychophysiological, Behavioral, and Cognitive Coping

Why, then, do some persons develop difficulties dealing with chronic pain, and not others? The effectiveness of individuals' cognitive, behavioral, and psychophysiological coping skills largely determine their adjustment to chronic pain. Often chronic pain patients either lack these pain coping skills (i.e., a "skill deficit") or fail to employ the appropriate coping skills even though they know them (i.e., an "activation deficit"). These coping skills are presumed to play a pivotal role in determining an individual's adaptation to chronic pain and are diagrammed accordingly on the left side of Figure 9-1.

Cognitive Coping Skills

Persons who can overcome debilitating chronic pain frequently display effective cognitive coping skills. They can problem-solve, finding alternative methods and solutions when needed. They are flexible and realistic in setting and adjusting goals. They appreciate working on clusters of minor goals as a way to achieve larger goals. They see themselves as personally responsible for making their lives better and believe they have or can acquire the necessary skills for such changes. They have hope.

In contrast, chronic pain patients who are trapped in the pain cycle typically do not employ the foregoing skills. Indeed, their coping style appears to be quite the opposite: they do not problem solve effectively, their goals and expectations are unrealistic and inflexible, and they often act as hopeless victims. Many of their cognitive deficits may be related to depression.[4]

Recall that a typical individual in chronic pain experiences diminished functioning in almost all areas of daily life (e.g., occupational, marital, sexual, and recreational functioning are all likely to be adversely affected). Attempts to resume activity may result mainly in accentuated pain, not desired goals. After repeated failures in attempts to obtain desired goals (including getting "well"), many individuals develop what some depression theorists call "learned helplessness"[5]. These individuals come to feel helpless and hopeless, believing that nothing they (or anyone else) can do will ever make any difference. They tend to take excessive self-blame for negative occurrences and deny responsibility for positive outcomes.

Unfortunately, such negative "cognitive distortions" tend to be global rather than specific, tainting a broad spectrum of beliefs about oneself, one's world, and one's future.[6] Attention is focused on the negative, especially pain. Regardless of their actions, family and friends may be perceived by the patient as unconcerned. The pervasive "why bother?" attitude diminishes motivation for virtually all activity, even those that had been enjoyable or would seem to hold promise for success. Even legitimate treatment gains may be dismissed as insignificant. Depression (including its somatic, affective, and cognitive components) thus sometimes results from, and almost invariably causes further deterioration of, the pain cycle.

Behavioral Coping Skills

Persons coping effectively with pain seem to possess several key behavioral skills. Foremost may be those interpersonal skills involved in effective utilization of social supports. Being able to share concerns, frustrations, and successes with others in a way that elicits positive support (and does not alienate) seems particularly important. Assertiveness, active listening, and negotiating skills also may be key ingredients. Successfully coping individuals can plan ahead and manage their time effectively. They are able to divide large tasks into manageable smaller parts and they reward themselves appropriately (i.e., for approximation or attainment of successes, not failure; for small as well as large task accomplishments). They have developed a range of recreational and personal interest areas in which they can achieve successes. Chronic pain patients trapped in the pain cycle seem to lack or fail to employ these skills.

Psychophysiological Coping Skills

One will frequently observe chronic pain patients bracing, guarding, limping, and/or posturing as they move about. Although these behaviors are often attempts to avert or control pain, they typically make the pain worse because of how they create excessive muscle tension. (Even though these behaviors are ineffective in controlling pain, they may continue because they elicit attention and sympathy from others.) Note that almost all emotions (including positive ones) can increase muscle tension and thereby increase pain. Persons who cope effectively with their pain are aware of and able to control their muscle tension levels. This may be a natural reaction or a result of training in relaxation procedures (e.g., EMG biofeedback, progressive muscle relaxation training, yoga, self-hypnosis, use of imagery). Although being able to relax in the prone position is useful, it seems particularly important (and difficult) for the chronic pain patient to learn to relax the musculature while being active.

A Healthy Adaptation-Disability Continuum

We have presented a model of chronic pain that addresses both conditioning and learning influences and the adequacy of an individual's psychophysiological, behavioral, and cognitive coping responses as critical factors in the prevention, development, and treatment of chronic pain. It is also important to note that adaptations to pain are believed to exist on a health/disability continuum with regard to each of these factors. This is illustrated in the far right panel of Figure 1. At the disability extreme are those individuals whose environment only rewards pain behaviors and ignores or punishes any attempted "well" (effective coping) behaviors. Indeed, such individuals usually either do not have (or do not employ) effective coping behaviors. Conversely, at the healthy extreme are individuals whose environment rewards "coping well" efforts. Even though pain persists, they employ effective coping responses. It is believed that as individuals' coping with chronic pain becomes entrenched maladaptively, they are moving on the continuum from relative health to relative disability. Essentially, the objective of behavioral chronic pain treatment programs is to reverse this process, by both enabling and appropriately rewarding movement toward healthy adaptation.

BEHAVIORAL ASSESSMENT AND TREATMENT

Behavioral Assessment

There are several methods that can be applied to evaluate patients' coping skills and adaptation to persistent pain. A *behavioral interview* is often quite helpful. One major purpose of the interview is to determine how patients spend their time during the day. Specific patterns of pain and well behavior are identified, and variables that control these behavior patterns are identified through careful questioning. Formats for behavioral interviewing have been described by Fordyce.[7] We find it helpful to gather information on: a) activity level (e.g., time spent up and out of bed each day), and the range of activities, particularly the patient's involvement in pleasure activities, b) the patient's belief about the cause of pain and the future trajectory of their pain, c) signs of depression (e.g., change in sleep or eating patterns, decreased energy, and libido), and d) changes in marital and family interactions that may be occurring.

A second approach to behavioral assessment is the use of *daily activity diaries*. Patients can be provided with simple diaries and asked to record time spent in activities such as sitting, standing or walking, and reclining as well as medication intake and ratings of pain severity. By examining these diaries, correlations between activity and medication intake may be examined. One common pattern is that patients may push themselves to continue an activity until their pain becomes intolerable and then rest or take pain medication. Another common finding is that pain may be increased during stressful periods of the day. Daily-activity diaries are particularly helpful when working with patients who are depressed because these patients tend to underestimate their activity and distort pain ratings as well. Patients often spontaneously remark that keeping a daily diary is a useful treatment procedure in and of itself.

A third approach to behavioral assessment is careful *observation* of the patient's behavior. These observations can be carried out at the end of a clinical interview by asking patients to walk or to shift from a reclining to a standing position since these behaviors tend to increase pain in most patients.[8] Behaviors such as guarded movement, rubbing or touching the painful area, and facial grimacing are easily observed and can be reliably recorded by trained observers. Standardized samples of pain behavior can also be gathered by having patients engage in a routine set of activities such as sitting, standing, walking, and reclining and recording the pain behaviors that occur. Behavioral observations can also be carried out during a physical examination or physical therapy evaluation. Observations of pain behavior are helpful in determining whether the level of pain behavior is excessive or not and also in examining whether the pain behavior is consistently related to factors that increase nociception such as movement. By watching patients' behavior in different settings, one can also determine how consistent the behavior is. Patients, for example, may appear to be in a significant amount of discomfort when discussing their pain with a consulting physician but appear to be quite comfortable one hour later when they are walking out of the hospital with spouse. Pain behaviors that are clearly linked to nociception are more consistent across different settings whereas inconsistencies in pain behavior often occur in patients who may have developed an operant pain pattern.

A variety of methods can be used to evaluate whether environmental factors might be related to the patient's problems in coping with pain. Interviews with the spouse and patient, observations of the patient when being visited by family, and careful analysis of daily activity diaries are often quite revealing. Spouse and family may support and encourage the patient to remain active and functional or they unwittingly may reinforce maladaptive pain behavior. Their response is a key factor affecting the patient's placement along the health-disability continuum discussed earlier. Solicitous responses take various forms such as the habit of bringing the patient pain medication, encouraging the patient to rest, or excusing the patient from unwanted family responsibilities. In many cases, the patient's spouse has learned to anticipate increased pain and actively discourages the patient from attempting social or vocational activities that he may be capable of. Alternatively, spouse or family members may become angry and resentful and begin to withdraw from the patient. When the patient seems to do well, the family may give him little attention whereas when his pain behavior becomes quite extreme, they "give in" and do attend to the patient.

Interviews with spouse and family often reveal that there are close relatives or friends who have had persistent pain or other chronic medical conditions. The patient may well have learned certain responses to pain or illness by observing these individuals. For example, the patient who was brought up by a parent who had chronic pain may very well learn some maladaptive responses such as an overreliance on rest or medication. Patients frequently turn to individuals in their social and cultural environment for suggestions on managing chronic pain or illness. In fact some patients rely more on the recommendations of friends and relatives than on treatment recommendations provided by physicians or medical personnel. Social and cultural mores obviously can play an important role in determining an individual patient's adaptation to chronic pain.

A final approach to behavioral assessment is *psychological testing*.[3] Data gathered with objective tests such as the Minnesota Multiphasic Personality Inventory (MMPI) or other standardized psychological tests are often utilized to evaluate how successfully the patient is coping with pain. High scores on scales measuring hypochrondriasis, depression, or hysteria typically indicate that the patient is coping poorly with pain and has more severe dysfunction in vocational, social, and marital spheres. Anxiety is often a core problem with these patients, and training in coping skills designed to reduce anxiety is indicated. Relaxation and biofeedback training often enables those patients to cope better with the cognitive and physiological correlates of anxiety. Patients who show elevations on scales measuring more severe psychopathology such as psychasthenia and schizophrenia usually have the most significant problems managing their pain and experience a high degree of psychological disturbance. The coping skills of these patients are quite poor, and most have long histories of emotional disturbance dating back to before the onset of pain. These patients have serious psychopathology and require ongoing psychiatric treatment to get any benefit from training in pain management techniques. With appropriate psychiatric treatment some of these patients are eventually able to develop good pain coping skills.

Behavioral Treatment

Behavioral treatment approaches to chronic pain have both immediate and long-term goals. Increasing activity level and decreasing narcotic medication usage are typically the primary initial targets. These goals are usually achieved by changing the reinforcement contingencies in the patient's environment so as to reward adaptive and not the maladaptive responses. The more global goal, however, is to enhance the individual's capacity to sustain an independent and satisfying life, one not necessarily free of pain, but one free of interference from pain. Achieving this broader goal entails development of appropriate cognitive, behavioral, and psychophysiological coping strategies. Moreover, it necessitates the patient's acceptance of personal responsibility for his well-being.

At the onset, however, many chronic pain patients are so depressed, enmeshed in the chronic pain cycle, and/or focused on obtaining a complete cure that they cannot or will not work effectively toward rehabilitative goals. While particularly difficult, such individuals are not completely hopeless. We find that contingency management treatment approaches often successfully begin the process toward healthy adaptation.

Contingency Management Approaches

The basic principle of contingency management approaches is realignment of the patient's reinforcers so that approaches toward improved function (and not pain behaviors) are consistently rewarded.[7] In our program this is accomplished primarily through a structured activity/rest program and time-contingent narcotic medication taper[1].

For the activity-rest program, we have patients engage in activity *and* rest an exact number of minutes each hour throughout the day. Gradually and systematically, the proportion of activity is increased. In this way, activity becomes independent of (rather than contingent upon) pain level, thereby breaking the pain cycle.

We begin by having patients record their current (baseline) level of activity for 1 to 2 days. They are instructed to record both "uptime" and "downtime" in minutes per hour. Normally downtime is defined as all time spent reclining (whether in bed, on a sofa, or in a reclining chair); uptime includes walking, standing, and sitting (each of which typically presents problems for chronic pain patients). Based on these records (verified by nurse observations) and the patient's own ability assessment, we establish with the patient an activity level (in minutes of uptime per hour) that is significantly below the current level and which we believe to be readily attainable *throughout* the waking day. We start most patients at approximately 20 to 30 minutes of uptime per hour, although 5 to 10 minutes per hour is common and 30 seconds per hour is not unheard of. With the most recalcitrant patients, nursing staff initially direct compliance with the program; otherwise, they simply monitor it. Each day the uptime goal is increased approximately 1 to 2 minutes for most patients.

Compliance with the activity-rest program (and utilization of other effective coping behaviors—defined above) is socially rewarded (with attention and praise) by members of the nursing staff and treatment team. Conversely, pain behaviors (e.g., moaning, limping, rubbing, bracing, grimacing) are given less attention and thus not socially rewarded as strongly.

The time-contingent medication taper is used because patients often enter the program dependent on narcotic analgesic medications. They typically take this medication on a PRN (as needed) basis, thereby creating quite variable analgesic levels in the body system and providing a strong reinforcer for pain signals. One of the program psychiatrists determines an appropriate baseline level (approximately current usage). This level of analgesic (often its methadone equivalent) is incorporated into a "pain cocktail" of cherry syrup delivered on a strict *time-contingent* schedule (every 6 hours) rather than contingent on pain complaints. Each day, the amount of analgesic is tapered. Although patients are told the general goal, they are not alerted to the specific amounts of medication in a given cocktail. Most patients are able to eliminate narcotic usage completely using this time-contingent pain cocktail method.[9]

Coping Skills Development

Patients are trained and guided in developing more effective cognitive, behavioral, and psychophysiological coping skills. This training is accomplished primarily through an individualized biofeedback program and behavior therapy group (The Pain Management Group), individual therapy to develop a home program, and a relapse prevention program.

Biofeedback. In the biofeedback program, patients are initially given daily instruction in progressive muscle relaxation. Their practice is guided by a 40-minute audiotape augmented by personalized instructions from a biofeedback technician. Training is enhanced with audio EMG biofeedback, normally from the frontalis or upper trapezius muscles. At this stage, learning and practice take place in a reclining position. Patients are given a copy of the audiotape and loaned a tape player with instructions to practice two or three times during the day. Basic relaxation skills are usually mastered within several days.[10]

Several steps are then taken to assist patients in actively utilizing relaxation in their daily environment. First, they are gradually weaned from the audiotaped instructions and are encouraged to practice shortening the time needed to achieve relaxation. We then introduce "mini-practice" exercises. Mini-practices involve a 30-second scanning of the muscles to determine areas of tension, followed by relaxation of any problem areas. To provide practice reminders we give patients a dozen small adhesive-backed dots to affix in prominent places in their room (on their telephone, mirror, etc.). This helps patients develop the habit of routinely checking tension levels (without first having to experience a pain cue). Patients are also trained in applied relaxation. Using a portable EMG biofeedback device, our biofeedback technicians next guide patients in utilizing their relaxation skills during sitting, standing, and (finally) movement. This last phase seems particularly important in helping patients reduce their anticipatory tension.

Pain Management Group. The Pain Management Group is a structured behavior therapy group that serves as the setting to help patients acquire behavioral and cognitive coping skills previously mentioned. The primary focus of the group is enabling patients to define, measure, and change daily activity patterns affected by pain using a variety of pain coping skills. To enhance their understanding and support of the program goals, spouses and family members are encouraged to attend these group sessions with patients. Patients typically participate in 10 1-hour sessions. Cognitive coping skill topics include utilizing distraction and imagery methods, recognizing self-defeating thoughts, and using rational coping statements. Behavioral skills include controlling pain through the activity-rest cycle, setting realistic activity goals, and dealing effectively with spouse and family responses. Psychophysiological topics include a primer on stress reactions and physiological arousal and the effects of deconditioning. During sessions, patients are encouraged to exchange creative problem solutions and to practice new skills where appropriate; any talk about individual pain is discouraged. Self-control is consistently emphasized by encouraging patients to make their own choices as to target problems, measurement methods, and treatment strategies. Because group membership is "open-ended," patients with more experience in the program frequently model appropriate skills and attitudes for newer patients. Importantly, each session concludes with a behavioral homework assignment (e.g., graph activity data, practice new cognitive coping strategies) that is reviewed during the next group session.

Home programs. One of the most important phases in treatment of the chronic pain patient is establishing a treatment program that can be carried out in the home setting following discharge. Setting up such a program requires that one closely work with both the patient and spouse. We encourage spouses to go through all treatment sessions with the patient during the final 2 days of admission. A conference is then set up with the patient and spouse to review ew the basic elements of the patient's home program.

It is helpful to begin planning for home programs by asking the spouse to comment on changes that he or she has noticed on the part of the patient. A spouse will often remark that the patient looks better, is much less anxious and irritable, and complains less of pain. During the discussion, patients usually remark that their progress is due in large part to their use of new pain management skills such as relaxation training or activity-rest cycling. The need to continue to apply these skills in the home setting is then reinforced by the therapist. The four basic elements of the home program are then described: 1) the daily program, 2) the flare-up plan, 3) goals for the next 2 months, and 4) "the *don't* list". Patient, spouse, and therapist work together to set up a home program that is uniquely suited to the patient's needs. Each element of the program is discussed in a frank and open manner, and criticism by the patient and spouse is encouraged. The goal is to develop a program that is both effective and practical.

Each patient's home program is written out on a home-program summary sheet. A copy is given to the patient, and a second copy is kept in the patient's file. The summary sheet lists each of the four major elements of the home program.

Daily program. Thedaily program consists of activities and techniques patients intend to use each day at home in order to manage their pain. A typical daily program, for example, might consist of the following: 1) practice with the relaxation tape—twice a day; 2) physical therapy exercises—twice a day; 3) activity-rest cycling—60 minutes up, 10 minutes, down; 4) work on a crafts or art project; and 5) take medication as prescribed. We ask the patient to describe each part of the daily program to the spouse. This helps clarify misconceptions that the patient may have and also helps the spouse become more familiar with the demands of the program. Patients are asked to identify particular times of the day for practice with relaxation or physical therapy. The spouse is also encouraged to try out the relaxation tape or become involved in a walking program as a way to reinforce compliance with the program.

The spouse is often confused about how to handle noncompliance. In the past, many spouses have become angry or oversolicitous because the patient does not seem to follow through on treatment recommendations. We encourage spouses to become involved in the patient's daily program in some way and thereby to increase attention paid appropriate behavior while at the same time minimizing the attention given when a patient fails to follow through with the daily program.

Flare-up plan. We inform all patients that they are likely to have a flare-up or increase in their pain on a temporary basis following discharge. Patients are provided with a behavioral plan to deal with this flare-up that is to replace their daily pain management program for a 3-day period. A typical flare-up plan includes the following: 1) change activity-rest cycling to decrease activity by 50 percent each hour; 2) over 3 days gradually increase activity to former level; 3) practice with relaxation techniques twice as often; 4) increase use of other cognitive pain-coping skills such as distraction, imagery, coping self-statements, or reinterpretation techniques; 5) cut back on physical therapy exercises as per instructions of physical therapist; 6) increase frequency of pleasant activities; and 7) inform spouse and family that flare-up plan is in progress. To maximize success, the spouse is encouraged to take an active role in implementation of the flare-up plan. We often use the analogy of a coach in a Lamaze childbirth preparation class. Like the coach, the spouse is encouraged to reinforce the patient for use of pain-coping skills, to be reassuring, and to be involved.

The flare-up plan has many psychological advantages. It prepares the patient and spouse both cognitively and behaviorally for a set-back. The flare-up is presented as a challenge to be dealt with, using learned pain-coping skills. Finally, the fact of increased pain is dealt with in a more open fashion by having patients admit that they are on a flare-up plan. This helps patients avoid the tendency to hide their pain and cycle to even higher levels of pain behavior before stopping. Follow-up sessions with patients and spouses indicate that this aspect of the home program is often the single most helpful element in the overall home program.

Goals for the next 2 months. Patients are asked to list a series of goals that they feel are realistically attainable within 2 months of discharge. Goals listed often include: 1) returning to church, 2) becoming involved in volunteer work, 3) beginning employment training, 4) returning to college, 5) increasing social activity, and 6) developing new hobbies or interests. Patients are told if the goals appear unrealistic and encouraged to select short-term goals that are more suited to their capabilities. Discussing these goals often provides an opportunity for patients to consider how they can apply elements of their daily program to new situations. Patients, for example, often are unsure as to how to use their activity-rest cycling when they are shopping in a mall or involved in volunteer work. Practical methods such as resting on a bench, going out to the car to recline, or bringing along a lawn chair recliner are discussed and evaluated by the patient and spouse. Anxieties about "looking different" or being rejected by others in social situations are identified, and methods to alleviate them are described.

"Don't" list. In the course of their inpatient treatment, patients often learn a number of activities that they should definitely avoid. These might include lifting more than 30 pounds, driving in an automobile for more than an hour, or walking more than 3 flights of stairs. Patients are encouraged to list these activities

on their home-program summary to ensure that they y and their spouse are clearly aware of these limitations. The need to change patterns of daily living, for example, to hire someone to help out with the heavy housework in order to have the patient stay within these limitations, can then be dealt with in a direct fashion.

Comment

We instruct patients to review their home program with every member of their family when they return home. They are told to place the home-program summary sheet in a public place such as near the calendar or on a cabinet door so that they can easily be reminded of it. We feel that asking patients to make a public commitment to their program helps greatly in enhancing compliance.

Relapse prevention program. Research indicates that the vast majority of chronic patients show improvements during treatment on specialized inpatient pain management units.[3] Follow-up studies conducted 1 to 5 years following treatment, however, indicate that 30 to 40 percent of patients may relapse. Most pain management programs are now incorporating methods to help prevent relapse. Two that we have found especially useful are telephone call follow-ups and the outpatient reinforcement group.

All patients in our program are seen for individual training in relaxation and biofeedback. They establish a working relationship with the biofeedback technician and, to enhance maintenance, we ask the technician to telephone the patient at regular intervals over the first year following discharge. The technician is provided with a checklist and asks the patient about compliance not only with relaxation techniques but all other aspects of their home program. A copy of the checklist is then provided to the Director of the Pain Management Program. Patients remark that they find this method of follow-up to be extremely beneficial. Most are surprised that they are actually called, and they report the calls do help them stay on their daily program. Telephone call follow-up sometimes reveals problems such as increased narcotic intake or major life stresses that make it hard for the patient to stay on the program. Recommendations for changes in the program can be made by the technicians, and the patient can also be encouraged to contact other staff members to alter the program as needed.

The outpatient reinforcement group is a 3-hour session that meets every 3 months and is open to all who have completed an inpatient course of treatment. The first hour of the group is a session for spouses only, and the final 2 hours are open to both patients and spouses. Topics in the groups are wide-ranging and determined by the participants. Patients typically request a review of flare-up programs. They comment both on their progress and failures. Signs of progress include return to work, going on a long vacation, staying off narcotics for an extended period of time, and becoming more involved in a variety of social activities. Patients often frankly describe what they perceive as failures in their program. One issue that has emerged consistently in these sessions has been the relationship of stress to increased pain and pain behavior. Most of these patients were initially reluctant to admit that stress related to their symptoms, but as they are followed over time, this relationship becomes more apparent.

One of the more interesting aspects of our outpatient reinforcement group is that following one of the first sessions, patients decided to begin a newsletter which they entitled *The Pain Chronicle*. The rationale was that the social support experienced during a group session was extremely beneficial, and patients desired a way to continue this support outside the group sessions. *The Pain Chronicle* is edited by two patients and the head nurse on the inpatient unit. The vast majority of contributors are patients, but sections have also been contributed by our physical therapists, biofeedback technicians, psychologists, and psychiatrists. Patients have submitted their own poetry, descriptions of trips they have taken, experiences they have had in managing their pain, recipes, and even cartoons. The patients are pleased with the product, and many have spontaneously remarked how helpful this newsletter is in reducing their sense of isolation and helplessness.

Conclusion

We have presented a behavioral assessment and treatment approach for chronic pain patients intended to put them on the road to a more healthy and functional adaptation to their disability. This approach has been successfully applied to many patients who had been unresponsive to other surgical and pharmacologic interventions. Unfortunately, we have also witnessed inpatient success washed away by an unchanged home environment (one responsive only to pain) and other social factors (such as disability status concerns). Careful follow-up seems essential.

For the clinician, the successes are often very dramatic and rewarding; be forewarned, however, that working with chronic pain patients—even within this behavioral framework—can be expected to be difficult, time-consuming, and very personally demanding.

References

1. Houpt JL, Keefe FJ, Snipes MT: The clinical specialty unit: The use of the psychiatry inpatient unit to treat chronic pain syndromes. *Gen Hosp Psychiat* 1984; 6: 65–70.
2. Follick MJ, Zitter RE, Ahern DK: Failures in the operant treatment of chronic pain. In Foa EB, Emmelkamp P (Eds), *Failures in Behavior Therapy*. New York; John Wiley & Sons, in press.
3. Keefe FJ: Behavioral assessment and treatment of chronic pain: Current status and future directions. *J Consult Clin Psych* 1982; 50: 896–911.
4. Lefebvre MF: Cognitive distortion and cognitive errors in depressed psychiatric and low back pain patients. *J Consult Clin Psych* 1981; 49: 517–525.
5. Abramson LY, Seligman MEP, Teasdale JD: Learned helplessness in humans: Critique and reformulation. *J Abnormal Psych* 1978; 87: 49–74.
6. Beck AT: *The Diagnosis and Management of Depression*. Philadelphia, University of Pennsylvania Press, 1967.

7. Fordyce WE: *Behavioral Methods for Chronic Pain and Illness.* St. Louis, C. V. Mosby, 1976.
8. Keefe FJ, Crisson JE, Snipes MT: Observational methods for assessing pain: A practical guide. In Blumenthal JA, McKee DC (Eds), *Applications in Behavioral Medicine and Health Psychology: A Clinician's Source Book.* Sarasto, FL, Professional Resource Exchange, in press.
9. France RD, Urban BJ, Keefe FJ: Long-term use of narcotic analgesics in chronic pain. *Soc Sci Med* 1984; 19: 1379–1382.
10. Keefe FJ, Schapira B, Williams RB, Brown C, Surwit RS: EMG-assisted relaxation training in the management of chronic low back pain. *Am J Clin Biofeedback* 1981; 4: 93–103.

Part III

SPELLS

Chapter 10

SEIZURES AND PSEUDOSEIZURES

J. Scott Luther, M.D.

Differentiation between real and pseudoepileptic seizures can be a complex, difficult problem; but sufficient information can be obtained from the history and a detailed description of the episodes to allow the practitioner to make an accurate assessment and diagnosis in the majority of cases. Episodes and spells are frequent problems faced by clinicians. In addition to clarifying distinguishing characteristics between real and pseudoepileptic seizures, it is hoped that this discussion will also provide a foundation and framework by outlining an approach to the patient with any type of spell or paroxysmal episode.

In order to recognize episodes that are most likely not epileptic in nature, one must appreciate the wide and varied clinical characteristics and expressions of real epileptic seizures. One logical method for approaching this understanding is by utilizing the current proposed international classification of epileptic seizures (Table 10-1).[1] This classification is important because of the etiologic, electroencephalographic, diagnostic, therapeutic, and prognostic implications that it carries for epilepsy in the general population.

The epilepsies are divided into two major categories—gen-

Table 10-1. Classification of Epileptic Seizures

I. GENERALIZED SEIZURES (bilaterally symmetrical and without local onset)
   A. Absences (petit mal)
   B. Tonic-clonic seizures (grand mal)
   C. Clonic seizures
   D. Tonic seizures
   E. Bilateral massive epileptic myoclonus
   F. Atonic seizures
II. PARTIAL SEIZURES (seizures beginning locally)
   A. Partial seizures with elementary symptomotology (generally without impairment of consciousness)
      1. with motor symptoms (includes Jacksonian seizures)
      2. with special sensory or somatosensory symptoms
      3. with autonomic symptoms
      4. compound forms
   B. Partial seizures with complex symptomatology (generally with impairment of consciousness)
      1. with impairment of consciousness only
      2. with cognitive symptomatology
      3. with affective symptomatology
      4. with "psychosensory" symptomatology
      5. with "psychomotor" symptomatology (automatisms)
      6. compound forms
   C. Partial seizures evolving to secondarily generalized seizures
      1. Simple partial evolving to generalized seizures
      2. Complex partial evolving to generalized seizures
      3. Simple partial evolving to complex partial evolving to generalized seizures
III. UNCLASSIFIED EPILEPTIC SEIZURES

eralized and partial. Conceptually generalized seizures, whatever the type, involve widespread if not total populations of both cortical and subcortical neurons simultaneously and synchronously. No localization for onset has been identified for this category of seizures. One popular hypothesis suggests that generalized seizures begin in deep midline subcortical generators and then recruit cortical neurons to result in the final clinical expression. Conversely, partial means *focal*. Partial seizures begin in a specific area of the brain and may remain very localized or may subsequently recruit other subpopulations of neurons to participate in the abnormal electrical discharge. When a sufficient population of neurons has been recruited and involved in the uncontrolled electrical discharge process which results in a clinical event that appears to be a generalized tonic-clonic seizure, this phenomenon is referred to as *secondary* as opposed to primary generalization. Frequently the focal onset of a patient's partial seizure may be so subtle that it goes unrecognized and the patients are not brought to clinical attention until they have had their first secondarily generalized seizure.

The generalized seizure disorders as a category have several characteristics which are entirely different from the partial seizure disorders. Primary generalized seizures tend to be diseases of childhood, whereas partial seizures begin at any age. Absence seizures typically begin between the ages of four and ten. The clinical expression of this type of seizure may be subtle or obvious. One of the more frequent subtle expressions is a dramatic decrease in school performance because the brief staring spells have been unrecognized—most lasting less than 5 seconds. The frequency is varied, but it is not unusual for these seizures to occur between 5 and 200 times a day. In addition, 30 percent of patients with absence will also have primary generalized tonic-clonic seizures at some point in time. The generalized tonic-clonic seizures which occur in patients with absence frequently occur during sleep and may bring the child to clinical attention. Primary generalized tonic-clonic seizures may also occur as a separate entity, again primarily in childhood. Another type of generalized seizure disorder has been more widely recognized in recent years chiefly because of the utilization of EEG/video monitoring. This seizure disorder is referred to by several different names—juvenile myoclonic epilepsy, juvenile epileptic myoclonus, or myoclonic epilepsy of Janz. Typically, these patients have a characteristic history of awakening in the morning and experiencing several myoclonic jerks of their extremities within a period of about 30 to 90 minutes after rising. It is not unusual for myoclonic jerks to occur for a period of 5 to 10 minutes, following which they will spontaneously subside. These patients usually come to clinical attention when the myoclonic jerks progress to the point that the patient finally experiences a generalized tonic-clonic seizure. Myoclonic jerks can also be a clinical component of absence, and therefore differentiation between absence and juvenile epileptic myoclonus is important. One major differentiation is the age of onset. Juvenile epileptic myoclonus usually begins later than absence, between the ages of eight to sixteen. The patients with juvenile epileptic myoclonus usually also have a more prominent myoclonic component which is more easily recognized from historical information. A point crucial to this discussion is that most medically intractable (uncontrolled by adequate anticonvulsant therapy) patients do not have one of the primary generalized epilepsies. The reasons are that 1) primary generalized epileptic seizures are the easiest to recognize in their usual form in the general population; 2) they are the category of seizure disorders which responds best to anticonvulsant therapy; and 3) only a small percentage of patients, if their diagnosis and treatment is correct, remain medically intractable and end up being referred to the medical center for further evaluation. The most common types of primary generalized seizure disorders that we see in the epilepsy center are adults who have had persistent absence seizures or patients who have juvenile epileptic myoclonus that is unresponsive to current anticonvulsant medications. The reason for the latter is that juvenile epileptic myoclonus had been poorly controlled with conventional anticonvulsants until the advent of valproic acid, the anticonvulsant of first choice in this disorder. Valproic acid is also the drug of choice for patients who have both absence and generalized tonic-clonic seizures. Although controversial, in absence without associated generalized tonic-clonic seizures ethosuximide remains the drug of first choice because of the potential hepatotoxicity of valproic acid. Generalized tonic-clonic seizures seem to respond well to any of the other major anticonvulsant drugs such as carbamazepine, phenytoin, phenobarbital, or primidone. In children and young females, carbamazepine is preferred by many epileptologists despite the expense, the necessity to follow blood work, and the need for multiple divided doses a day. Phenytoin has the potential for causing dysmorphic features in the form of gum hyperplasia and darkening of body hair which are unpopular side effects with children and young women. Phenobarbital and primidone have sedative side effects which may affect learning behavior.

By contrast, partial seizures are the most difficult to control with anticonvulsant medications. Again, I want to emphasize that partial means *focal*. Partial seizures are subcategorized into simple or elementary, and complex. The way these are differentiated is on the basis of whether or not the patient loses the ability to process information or loses the ability to interact properly with the environment around him during the episode. Frequently, this is referred to as "loss of consciousness," which I feel is an incorrect term because it implies a dramatic clinical event such as falling to the ground, generalized motor activity, or bodily harm. Many partial seizures which do not secondarily generalize do not have as their clinical expression significant dramatic motor components. Most frequently, patients who are having complex partial seizures will exhibit confusion in the form of being unable to respond appropriately, or to remember, process, or retain information that is presented during the episode. By definition then, a patient with elementary or simple partial seizures will be able to process and retain information which is presented to him during an episode no matter what the clinical behavioral expression of the seizure is.

Behavior commonly seen during complex partial seizures consists of inappropriate staring into space, mumbling, swallowing or lip smacking, chewing, wringing of the hands, or fumbling with clothes or bed linens. Directed violence during a complex partial seizure is extremely rare.

Elementary partial seizures are most commonly manifested by motor behavior, such as the rhythmic jerking of one extremity or portion thereof; but occasionally patients will have complex motor behavior, such as posturing of both upper extremities or the entire body, and yet retain the ability to process information. The ability to vocalize and thus speak is frequently impossible during the episode but they still retain their ability to remember.

Why then this emphasis on partial seizures? In any population of epileptic patients, including all age groups, the most common type of seizure that occurs is complex partial. About 45 percent of an epileptic population will have as its major seizure type, or the predominant seizure type, complex partial seizures. In a population of patients above the age of eighteen to twenty who have had a new seizure onset, the percentage with complex partial seizures jumps to around 75 to 80 percent; thus adults with new onset seizures that are not related to metabolic disorders such as renal failure, alcohol withdrawal, hypoglycemia, etc., have a 75 to 80 percent chance of complex partial seizures as their seizure type. What complicates issues even more is that approximately 60 percent of patients who have complex partial seizures will at some time during their epileptic history exhibit secondarily generalized seizures that bring the patient to clinical attention. When such secondarily generalized seizures are captured in the laboratory using EEG/video monitoring, they invariably begin as complex partial seizures and then evolve to generalized tonic-clonic activity. The partial seizures are the most difficult to control. As was noted earlier, primary generalized seizures are the easiest to control with proper anticonvulsant medications, are primarily a disease of childhood, and carry the best prognosis. Unlike the primary generalized seizures that begin in childhood, partial seizures, elementary or complex, may begin at any age. There is a bimodal distribution in epileptic populations when partial seizures tend to have their highest incidence. The first peak is between adolescence and the early twenties, with the second after the age of fifty-five. In any group of patients with complex partial seizures, approximately 15 percent will remain medically intractable: that is, they will not have adequate control, no matter in what combination nor how many anticonvulsants they are on. These are the patients who should come to evaluation for possible surgical intervention.

With this background information on real epileptic seizures, several criteria become helpful in trying to distinguish pseudoseizures from real seizures (Table 10-2).[2] It should be emphasized that each individual criterion is not mutually exclusive for representing either an epileptic or behavioral event.[3,4,5] Both real and pseudoseizures tend to be paroxysmal or sudden in onset. Real epileptic seizures characteristically are stereotyped in nature: the patient exhibits the same repetitive behavior with each episode that occurs. Most complex partial seizures and other real seizures last between 15 seconds and 5 minutes, as opposed to

Table 10-2. Useful Criteria in the Evaluation of Seizures and Spells

A. Age of onset of each spell type
B. Frequency of each type
C. Precipitating factors
D. Auras or prodromes
E. Occur alone?
F. Occur in sleep?
G. Associated loss of consciousness or confusion
H. Tongue biting
I. Incontinence
J. Self-injury
K. Directed rage
L. Response to medication
M. Postevent somnolence

pseudoepileptic seizures, which may be more prolonged. Brief episodes are more difficult to distinguish as being real or behavioral than more prolonged ones, because most patients have recovered from their real epileptic seizures in 20 to 30 minutes. On the other hand, behavioral motor activity that lasts from a half hour to hours is more likely to fall in the pseudoepileptic category.

EEGs may be very helpful but also may be misleading. A small percentage of any normal population has an abnormal EEG and yet has never experienced any known seizure activity. Even more complicating is analysis in the inheritable seizure disorder group. For instance, 30 to 50 percent of the sibs of a patient who is having clinical absence will have spike wave discharges on their EEGs and yet will have never had a clinical seizure. Therefore the interictal or interevent EEG is of only limited value for distinguishing real from behavioral events.[5] The hardest EEG criteria that can be used in establishing the diagnosis of a pseudoepileptic seizure are reproductions of the patient's typical clinical episode while under continuous EEG/video monitoring. If there is no background alteration in the EEG prior to, during, or following the episode, this would favor the event's being pseudoepileptic in nature.[5]

Several words of caution need to be mentioned here. First, most patients with elementary partial seizures do not have scalp EEG changes during their ictal events; and second, EEG criteria alone should not exclusively be used to make a decision as to whether a patient's clinical event represents a real seizure or a behavioral phenomenon. Thus, in many cases, firsthand observation or videotape analysis must be used to confirm the clinical characteristics of the episode. This becomes particularly important with the more widespread use of ambulatory EEG. A number of patients have been seen in this epilepsy center who have been diagnosed as having pseudoepileptic seizures and who did not have scalp EEG changes during their events. When these patients' events were eventually captured on videotape, analysis revealed a number were having elementary partial seizures. Therefore, videotape is used to confirm the clinical characteristics and also to clarify whether or not the event captured is indeed representative of the patient's typical clinical events. Review of the videotape by a reliable nonpatient observer frequently will aid in confirmation. The reproduction of behavior in the laboratory that is not typical for the patient's clinical behavior should not be considered of any diagnostic significance. Thus, the clinical history actually becomes one of the most important tools in determining whether a patient has real seizures or pseudoseizures.

In gathering historical information, it is critical to try to obtain a description of the patient's episodes from a reliable firsthand observer. The time and energy expended in doing so may precisely clarify the nature of the patient's clinical events and obviate the need for extensive laboratory studies or unwarranted medication therapy. In reference to spells or episodes, it is very important to determine how many different kinds of spells a patient has and whether or not they are all the same (stereotyped), or whether the reliable observer recognizes subtle or major differences in the various types of episodes. Other important criteria are whether the events represent variations on a theme or whether the observer recognizes different events as distinct clinical entities. For instance, the patient with complex partial seizures usually begins or "goes into" his seizure the same way every time. Occasionally such patients may exhibit secondarily generalized tonic-clonic seizures; but it is important to know whether those seizures began with the patient's typical complex partial seizure. Conversely, it is important to know whether the patient falls down and strikes his head or beats with his extremities in one episode and yet exhibits entirely different behavior in other episodes.

There are other criteria that aid in distinguishing pseudoepileptic from real seizures. The age of onset of each type of episode is significant. This becomes most important in patients who are having both real seizures and pseudoepileptic seizures.[3,4,5,6] The pseudoepileptic seizures most frequently represent the patient's most current or most recent behavioral episodes. Frequency is also very telling. Multiple daily or weekly episodes of recent onset in the setting of a normal EEG should raise the suspicion that these might be behavioral in nature. Frequently, patients who have pseudoepileptic seizures will recognize emotional precipitating factors such as anger or fear. It is also of consequence whether the events occur when the patient is alone, if they occur during sleep, if there is loss of consciousness or confusion, and if they have been associated with any significant trauma. Urinary incontinence had been considered a strong criterion in support of an event representing real epileptic seizure; however, there are now several studies where up to 5 to 10 percent of patients with pseudoepileptic seizures experience urinary incontinence during their events.[6] Fecal incontinence has not been reported during pseudoepileptic seizures. Directed rage, which we define as unprovoked behavior during the event, that can be interpreted in no fashion other than infliction of physical harm on an individual or inanimate object, is extremely rare during real epileptic seizures. For instance, throwing furniture through windows, beating one's spouse, or assaulting someone with a weapon is not considered epileptic behavior.

In contrast to prior thinking and ideas, three independent studies in patients with pseudoseizures do not substantiate the notion that most pseudoepileptic seizures occur in patients with real seizures.[4,5,7] These studies all indicate that only about a third or less of patients with pseudoepileptic seizures have ever had real seizures. Response to medication does offer some discrimination, but again, caution against developing a false sense of security is warranted. As mentioned earlier, 15 percent of patients with real complex partial seizures will not have adequate control of their seizures, regardless of the combination or adequacy of anticonvulsant medications.

Other characteristics of the patient's behavioral events are useful in discriminating between behavioral and real seizures. This is nothing new, as evidenced by the writings of Gowers in 1890 (Table 10-3).[4] Analysis of this table will reveal many of the discriminating variables already discussed in reference to pseudoepileptic seizures, such as the onset being gradual and precipitated by emotion. Screaming or yelling throughout an event is very characteristic of pseudoepileptic seizures. Patients also frequently exhibit generalized rigidity, with struggling behavior often associated with opisthotonus. This classic posturing with exaggerated arching of the back is distinctly unusual in real epileptic seizures. The motor activity seen is often asynchronous and although it may be coordinated from one side of the body to another, often it will not show a definitive pattern.

In a group of 30 patients with pseudoseizures studied at Duke, 15 were having a single type of episode that was pseudoepileptic in nature. The remaining 15 patients were having two or more types of episodes, and in 12 of these patients, both types were found to represent pseudoepileptic seizures. Disturbingly, two patients had three and one patient actually had four types of events which all turned out to be pseudoepileptic in nature.[5] Nineteen of these patients were having these episodes at a frequency higher than one per day. Only five of the patients reported being alone when their pseudoepileptic events occurred and one reportedly occurred during sleep. Although three patients stated they had had urinary incontinence during their episodes, this was not reproduced in the laboratory. We have, however, observed the phenomenon of urinary incontinence in pseudoepileptic seizures since this group was reported. No fecal incontinence was seen. Self-injury was reported by five patients. Over 93 percent of the patients were on anticonvulsant medication, with nine patients on single drug therapy and the remainder on two or more medications. Characteristically, the clinical features, the frequency of occurrence, and the duration

Table 10-3. Comparison of Features of Nonepileptic and Epileptic Seizures (After Gowers)

	Nonepileptic	Epileptic
Precipitant cause	Emotion	Usually none
Warning	Palpitation, malaise, choking, distraction	Any, especially unilateral sensory or epigastric aura
Onset	Often gradual	Sudden
Scream	During course	At onset, if any
Convulsion	Rigidity or struggling	Rigidity followed by jerking (tonic-clonic), rarely rigidity alone
Tonic posture	Often opisthotonic	Partial flexion
Body movements	No definite pattern	Definite sequence, each seizure similar
Head movements	Often side to side	To one side, rarely side to side
Biting	Lips, arms, other people, things	Tongue
Micturation	Very infrequent	Frequent
Defecation	Never	Occasional
Talking	Frequent, calling names	Rare
Duration	More than 5 minutes, often much longer	A few minutes
Restraint necessary	To control violence	To prevent injury
Termination	Spontaneous or induced (pressure, suggestion, cold water)	Spontaneous

of symptoms were unmodified by this anticonvulsant therapy. Real epileptic seizures were determined to occur in only nine patients. Half of the baseline EEGs were abnormal. The patients were subsequently monitored and analysis of all the characteristics revealed the nature of their behavioral events.

In conclusion, the differentiation between real epileptic and pseudoseizures may be difficult, but with a detailed history and the framework of the currently proposed international seizure classification, a correct diagnosis can be made in many cases. Any clue to the correct diagnosis may be helpful. When the Duke Center for the Advanced Study of Epilepsy reviewed its experience with real seizures, we found that the most common seizures seen were absence and complex partial. In contrast, behavior that mimicked primary generalized tonic-clonic seizures and elementary partial seizures which then evolved to secondarily generalized seizures were the most common seizure types seen in the pseudoepileptic group. For pseudoepileptic seizures behaviorally to mimic complex partial seizures is extremely rare. Frequent generalized seizure behavior that is unresponsive to medication is the most constant feature of pseudoepileptic seizures. For practical purposes, patients with frequent seizures or episodes of recent onset unaltered by anticonvulsants with a normal EEG should be particularly suspect for having pseudoepileptic seizures. The bottom line is "all that glitters is not gold, all that shakes and trembles doesn't need anticonvulsants." The distinction at times can be extremely difficult and may require in-depth analysis with simultaneous EEG/video monitoring for clarification.

References

1. Dreifuss FE, Bancaid J *et al:* Proposal for revised clinical and electroencelphalographic classification of epileptic seizures. *Epilepsia* 1981; 22:489–501.
2. Gowers WR: *Epilepsy and Other Chronic Convulsive Diseases: Their Cause, Symptoms and Treatment.* New York, Dover Publications, 1964.
3. Gulick TA, Spinks IP, King DW: Pseudoseizures: Ictal phenomena. *Neurol* 1982; 32:24–30.

4. King DW, Gallagher BB *et al:* Pseudoseizures: Diagnostic evaluation. *Neurol* 1982; 32:18–23.
5. Luther JS, McNamara JO *et al:* Pseudoepileptic seizures: Methods and video analysis to aid diagnosis. *Ann Neurol* 1982; 12:458–462.
6. Cohen RJ, Suter C: Hysterical "seizures"—Suggestion as a provocative EEG test. *Ann Neurol* 1982; 11:391–395.
7. Lesser RP, Lueders H, Dinner DS: Evidence for epilepsy is rare in patients with psychogenic seizures. *Neurol* 1983; 33:502–504.

Chapter 11

PANIC ATTACKS

J. Trig Brown, M.D.

In few of the psychomedical disorders is there as much excitement in the 1980s as in panic attacks. Advances are rapidly being made in understanding the pathophysiology of panic attacks and therapeutic modalities are being successfully applied. This chapter discusses the clinical picture, reviews our understanding of the etiology, and outlines approaches to diagnose and treat panic attacks.

Because panic attacks can occur in all Anxiety Disorders, one needs some knowledge of these states to fully understand panic attacks (Table 11-1). The three Anxiety Disorders are separated into those characterized by phobic behavior (Phobic Disorders), those primarily characterized by anxiety (Anxiety States), and those representative of pathological reactions to traumatic events (Post-Traumatic Stress Disorder or PTSD).[1]

The Phobic Disorders are divided into three classes: agoraphobia, the fear of being in a crowd or, paradoxically, of being alone; social phobia, the fear of behaving in an embarassing or humiliating manner in public; and the simple phobias, fears of discrete objects. The Anxiety States are similarly divided into three classes: panic disorder, the anxiety state characterized by

Table 11-1. The Anxiety Disorders

Anxiety Disorders

1. Phobic Disorders
   - agoraphobia
   - social phobia
   - simple phobia

2. Anxiety States
   - panic disorder
   - generalized anxiety
   - obsessive-compulsive

3. Post-Traumatic Stress Disorder

panic attacks; the generalized anxiety disorders, the new terminology for what was once known as anxiety neurosis; and the obsessive compulsive disorder, characterized by obsessions and compulsive behavior. The third Anxiety Disorder is the Post-Traumatic Stress Disorder, a pathological (often delayed) reaction to an event that would be stressful to most individuals. Examples include a natural disaster, a prisoner-of-war or other wartime experiences, or significant losses.

Figure 11-1 schematically represents the effects that panic attacks have on the individual. When the spontaneous fear and apprehension of a panic attack is sensed, one normally tries to escape the situation. This is called escape behavior. After repeated panic attacks, one develops anticipatory anxiety that one will experience a panic attack. If this anticipatory anxiety is of such a degree that it starts limiting the person's behavior, then phobic behavior has developed. In other words, phobic behavior develops when the individual starts avoiding situations that have been associated with the panic attacks. This interaction between the panic attack and the anticipatory anxiety is important when evaluating patients and when planning therapy.

```
        panic
        attack
       ↙     ↘
escape          
behavior  ←——  anticipatory
(phobias)       anxiety
```

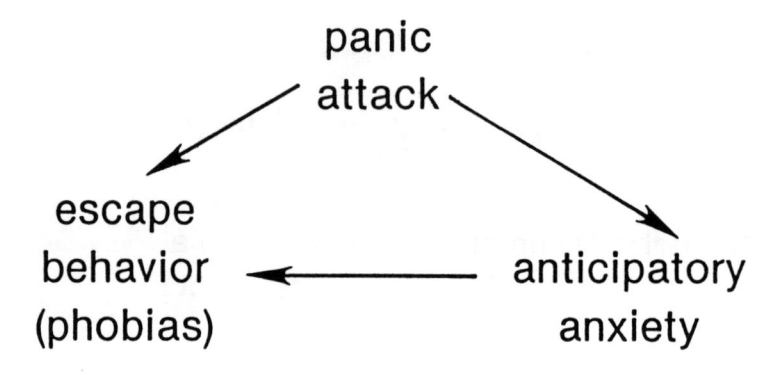

Figure 11-1. **Effects panic attacks have on the individual.**

CLINICAL PICTURE

Panic attacks are defined as spontaneous, periodic episodes of apprehension and fear. Patients often have difficulty describing the symptoms which affect most systems of the body (Table 11-2). Patients may have primarily cardiopulmonary symptoms with dyspnea, palpitations, chest pain, choking, or a smothering

Table 11-2. **Manifestations of Panic Attacks**

Panic Attacks
manifestations

dyspnea	paresthesias
palpitations	hot and cold flashes
chest pain	sweating
choking, smothering	faintness
dizziness, vertigo, or unsteadiness	trembling, shaking
feeling of unreality	fear of dying, going crazy, losing control

sensation. The symptoms can be more those of a neurologic nature; for example, dizziness, vertigo, unsteadiness, or feelings of unreality. Not infrequently patients will describe paresthesias, hot and cold flashes, sweating, faintness, trembling, and shaking. Some patients have more cognitive manifestations and notice primarily the fear of dying, going crazy, or losing control.

Patients may have some of these symptoms, or all. Patients who have few, or whose symptoms are primarily in one organ system account for the historical difficulty in grasping an understanding of panic attacks. For example, if a patient goes to a cardiologist complaining primarily of chest pain or palpitations, he may be labelled as having Da Costa's syndrome, irritable heart, cardiac neurosis, or effort syndrome, after an extensive negative workup. On the other hand, if they present with dizziness, unsteadiness, and paresthesias to a neurologist, they may be labelled as having vertigo hysterique. The pulmonologist may see the patients primarily with shortness of breath and may be most impressed with the hyperventilation syndrome. All of these terms have been used in the literature to describe what we now call panic attacks.

Panic attacks have a prevalence of 2 to 5 percent in the general population.[2] In persons who use medical care, specifically those at a cardiology subspeciality, up to 10 to 15 percent of these patients have panic attacks. There is a female preponderance (65 to 80 percent) and the age of onset is usually in the late teens, twenties, or early thirties. Patients have been seen with the onset of their panic attacks after age sixty-five, but this is unusual. A marked familial predilection for this disorder exists, 20 to 30 percent of the first degree relatives of patients with panic attacks also have them.

ETIOLOGY

The etiology of panic attacks remains unknown, although in this area much progress has been made. In 1871, Dr. J.M. Da Costa described over 200 soldiers seen while working as a military physician.[3] These men were between the ages of sixteen and twenty-five and complained primarily of palpitations. Other symptoms noted were giddiness, "cardiac pain," "oppression upon exertion," headache, disturbed sleep, excessive sweating, and a variety of gastrointestinal symptoms. These symptoms are strikingly similar to those described above in patients with panic attacks (Table 11-2). These soldiers had a good prognosis when removed from the combat situation. Da Costa hypothesized that, due to an overactivity of the sympathetic nervous system, these soldiers' hearts had become irritable. This was the first attempt at explaining panic attacks.

The next landmark in understanding the etiology of panic attacks involves lactate. In the 1940s it was observed that patients with anxiety attacks had a greater rise in serum lactate after exercise than did a group of controls. That finding was buried d in the literature for about 20 years until Pitts and McClure performed the first lactate infusion experiment.[4] In 14 patients with panic attacks and 10 control patients, they infused sodium lactate in a double-blinded fashion. In 13 of 14 patients and in only 2 of 10 controls panic attacks were precipitated. This experiment has been reproduced with similar findings by a number of investigators, although the explanation of this fascinating phenomena is not clear.

Currently investigators are focusing on the locus ceruleus, that neuroanatomical structure at the base of the fourth ventricle.[5] In experimental animals, if one stimulates the locus ceruleus, behavior that resembles that of a fearful animal is produced. On the other hand, if one ablates or blocks the locus ceruleus's activity with drugs, this behavior is attenuated. It appears now that the locus ceruleus is close to the final common pathway for the expression of panic.

Figure 11-2 schematically represents a model for understanding the etiology of panic attacks. The locus ceruleus, near the final common pathway for expressing panic, seems to have a threshold for firing. Exact modulators of this threshold are not known and in fact many factors may influence it. The genetic makeup of the individual, the person's development, stresses, illnesses, and losses may all influence the threshold for expressing panic attacks and hence contribute to the episodic and varied clinical course of panic states.

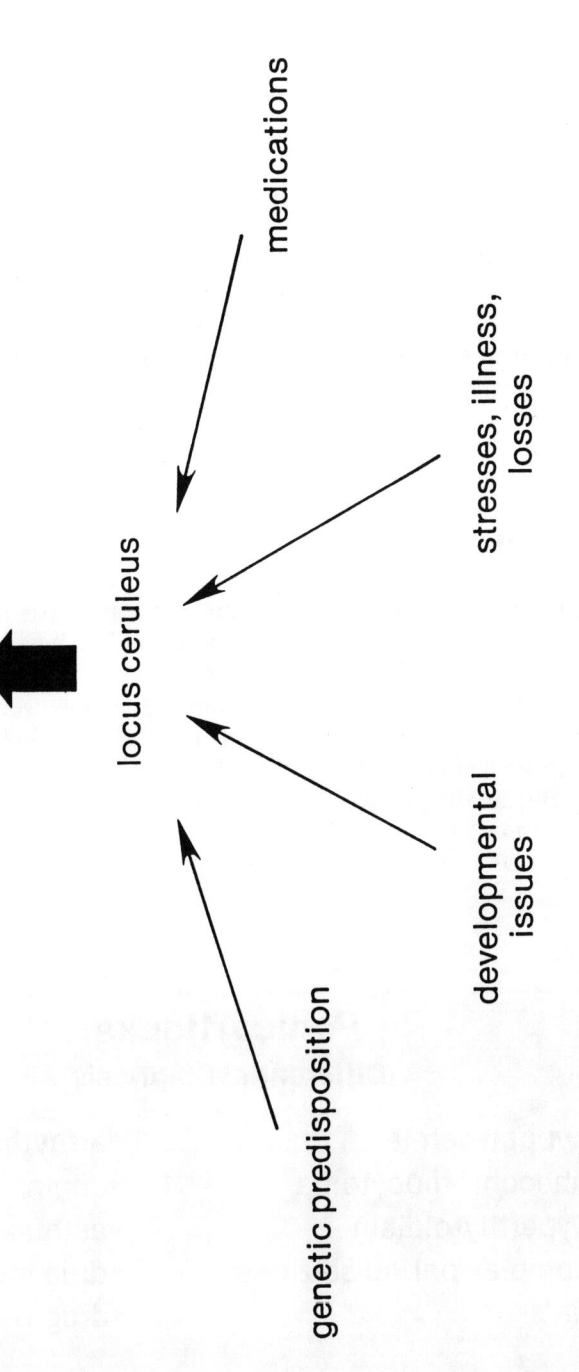

Figure 11-2. A multifactorial model of panic attacks.

Differential Diagnosis

The differential diagnosis of these symptoms is lengthy (Table 11-3). Essentially, any clinical situations that result in episodic symptoms, especially those of sympathetic overactivity, should be included in the differential. It is obvious that hypoglycemia, pheochromocytoma, and hyperthyroidism manifest autonomic overactivity and should be considered. Other episodic events associated with sympathetic overactivity include complex partial seizures, TIAs, arrhythmias, angina, asthma, and pulmonary emboli. Drug intoxication (over-the-counter sympathomimetics, caffeine, cocaine, or amphetamines) and drug withdrawal states (alcohol, barbiturates, and possibly benzodiazepines) should also be included.

Table 11-4 outlines one approach to evaluate these patients. On the left hand column are maneuvers and tests that should probably be done on all patients suspected of having panic attacks. During the history, particular attention should be paid to the nature of their spell, the circumstances they were in at the time, the relationship to meals or drugs; and, if possible, a witness of the spell should be interviewed.

During the physical exam, focus should be on the vital signs, cardiovascular exam, and neurologic exam. The most helpful bedside test when suspecting panic attacks is to hyperventilate

Table 11-3. Differential Diagnosis of Panic Attacks

Panic Attacks
Differential Diagnosis

- hypoglycemia
- pheochromocytoma
- hyperthyroidism
- complex partial seizures
- tia's
- arrhythmias
- angina
- asthma, embolus
- drug intoxication
- drug withdrawal

Table 11-4. Evaluation of Panic Attacks

Panic Attacks
Evaluation

- history
- physical
- hyperventilation
- hemoglobin
- thyroid panel

- 5 hour GTT
- urine catechols
- sleep EEG
- Holter monitor

the patient. If one can exactly reproduce their spell with hyperventilation, the diagnosis of panic attack is strongly supported. Often reproducing the spell with hyperventilation has a profound impact upon the patient and family. Most of these patients have seen many physicians worrying about a cardiovascular or a neurologic problem. When they see that they can reproduce these symptoms voluntarily through hyperventilation, the anticipatory anxiety is lessened.

The tests on the right-hand side of Table 11-4 are used more selectively. If the patients' symptoms are in any way meal-related or food-relieved, or if they have had any prior GI surgery, a 5-hour glucose tolerance test is indicated to exclude reactive hypoglycemia. If symptoms are suggestive of a pheochromocytoma (excessive sweating, tachycardia, or palpitations and headache) or if patients are tachycardiac or hypertensive with orthostatic hypotension, urine catecholamines should be measured. If the spells awaken the patient, if a witness describes behavior that sounds as if it could possibly be a seizure, or if an accident happened during the spells, an electroencephalogram should be obtained. At most institutions a sleep EEG with nasopharyngeal leads is used first in excluding complex partial seizures. Finally, if the patient is of an older age group or has a number of cardiovascular risk factors, ambulatory cardiac monitoring can best exclude an arrhythmia as a cause for the symptoms.

Treatment

Panic attacks respond well to a number of pharmacologic agents but, if one does just that, the patient may be left with phobic behavior or anticipatory anxiety (Figure 11-1). Table 11-5 outlines the therapeutic modalities successful in treating patients with panic attacks. For the panic attack itself imipramine remains a first-line treatment. Most of these patients are young, have normal cardiovascular systems, and tolerate this drug very well. In contrast to the MAO inhibitors, no dietary changes are needed with imipramine. Generally one starts with a low dose (25 mg at bedtime) and gradually increases the imipramine up to 150 to 200 mg at night. The goal is to completely abolish the panic attacks.

MAO inhibitors, the second group of drugs, are equal in effectiveness to imipramine. As mentioned before, dietary restrictions must be made while using this group of drugs. A third drug that is becoming more and more popular in treating panic and may some day replace imipramine as the treatment of choice

Table 11-5. Therapeutic Modalities for Panic Attacks

Panic Attacks
Treatment

Panic Attack	imipramine MAO-inhibitors alprazolam
Anticipatory Anxiety	psychotherapy benzodiazepines
Phobic Avoidance	behavioral therapies

is alprazolam. This new triazolobenzodiazepine has few side effects and therapeutically lessens both the anticipatory anxiety and the panic attacks. The doses of alprazolam required to abolish panic attacks are higher than the normal anxiolytic doses of this drug, some report using from 4 to 9 mg of alprazolam daily. The anticipatory anxiety also must be addressed. Benzodiazepines help, especially when coupled early in treatment with drugs more specific to the panic attacks. The patients need to be seen in some type of supportive relationship frequently with adjustments in medication made depending upon both side effects and benefits. If the patient has developed any phobic behavior, some of the more formal behavioral therapies will be necessary parts of the overall management plan. The major point in therapy must be reemphasized: treatment should be multidimensional, aimed at the panic attack, the anticipatory anxiety, and the phobic behaviors. Only in this way will these "complicated medical patients" be cured.

REFERENCES

1. Brown JT, Mulrow CD, Stoudemire, GA: The anxiety disorders. *Ann Intern Med* 1984; 100:558–564.
2. Sheehan DV: Current concepts in psychiatry: Panic attacks and phobias. *NEJM* 1982; 307:156–158.
3. Da Costa, JM: On irritable heart, a clinical study of a form of functional cardiac disorder and its consequence. *Am J Med Sci* 1871; 121:2–52.
4. Pitts, FN, Jr, McClure JN, Jr: Lactate meatolism in anxiety neurosis. *NEJM* 1967; 277:1329–1336.
5. Hoehn-Saric R: Neurotransmitters in anxiety. *Arch Gen Psychiatry* 1982; 39:735–742.

Part IV

FACTITIAL DISEASES

Chapter 12

PSYCHOCUTANEOUS SYNDROMES

Claude S. Burton, M.D.

Unlike the majority of psychosomatic illnesses, cutaneous diseases cannot be imagined. All patients presenting with factitial skin conditions will have lesions clearly visible on the skin (Table 12-1). The very nature of the traumatic process required to produce these lesions makes unconscious participation unlikely, excepting perhaps psychogenic pruritus or trauma to the skin that might theoretically occur while asleep, in a trance, or under the influence of a split personality.[1,2] With psychocutaneous syndromes the physician has the advantage. Diagnosing factitial skin disease in a patient with very obvious lesions is often much simpler than the evaluation of psychosomatic chest pain, headache, abdominal pain, and the like, where symptoms may be imaginary and objective signs are lacking. Imagination alone may sustain persistent abdominal pain or chest pain, but imagination alone will not sustain cutaneous gangrene.

By and large, patients with factitious skin disease are not as sophisticated as patients with factitious fever, endocrinopathy, coronary artery disease, or other maladies. To feign the latter, patients must be rather knowledgeable about the disease they are trying to simulate to convince the physician they are ill.

**Table 12-1.
Common Patterns of Factitial Dermatoses**

1. Ulcers and gangrenous lesions
2. Excoriations
3. Amputations
4. Purpura
5. Blisters
6. Ligatures

Therefore, patients with these illnesses are heavily represented by nurses and other health care workers.[3] The information and necessary means to feign thyrotoxicosis, hypoglycemia, hematuria, or fever are easily available and such illnesses lend themselves to artifactual mimicry.[4,5] While very little skill is required to injure the skin, to accurately mimic true cutaneous pathology is extraordinarily difficult even for the professional. No one, despite extensive research, has been successful at artificially creating psoriasis. Though spotting factitial lesions may challenge the best of dermatologists, our most reliable tool is knowledge of the spectrum of genuine cutaneous disease. Knowing the genuine makes it easier to recognize the phony.

Factitious lesions appear commonly in the field of dermatology. Each of us who has ever seen a factitial dermatosis is constantly on guard for this possibility. More difficult than making the diagnosis is determining the method the patient uses to produce the condition; and more difficult still is management of this occasionally devastating illness. For the uninitiated, a review of this fascinating problem will establish the appropriate index of suspicion.

CLASSIFICATION

Since each patient with factitious skin disease is unique, any classification serves to benefit the author more than the patient. For the purpose of this discussion I will divide patients with factitial dermatoses into three broad categories; malingerers, self-mutilators, and pickers and scratchers. To best define these subsets I will illustrate them by fictitious examples.

Case Number 1: Malingering Skin Disease

Mr. W. is a thirty-six-year-old male veteran drafted during the Vietnam conflict. During his tour of active duty he developed an episode of palpable purpura that on biopsy was consistent with leukocytoclastic vasculitis. Transfer back to the States was arranged to further study the possibility that this might represent a systemic vasculitis. Extensive evaluation failed to show renal, hepatic, pulmonary, gastrointestinal, or other involvement and the purpura gradually faded. Prior to his release, he developed such massive swelling in both hands that he was unable to make a fist. He was honorably discharged with a diagnosis of undefined connective tissue disease and placed on 100 percent Service-connected disability. At the time I first saw him approximately 8 years later, he continued to receive $1400 a month in tax-free disability income. Over that interval his case had been reviewed on a number of occasions and, because of persistent hand swelling, disability payments continued. In support of his claim was a large collection of photographs his wife had taken of his massively swollen, often purplish, hands. In fact, by mailing these to the review board he was able to document ongoing disability, thus avoiding periodic reexamination. The vasculitis had never returned and no laboratory abnormality was ever discovered, despite several exhaustive evaluations. On careful examination, the etiology was obvious. Ligature marks at the margins of the edema clearly established the cause of his swollen hands.

Mr. W. illustrates the features of factitial dermatoses in general and cutaneous malingering in particular (Table 12-2). The motives here are obvious. His condition resulted in removal from an unpleasant environment (active military duty) and provided handsome monetary rewards to boot. One must explore such considerations in every patient evaluated for chronic illness.[6] Where gain does not exist, one cannot make a strong case for simple malingering.

A true illness or injury often precedes the feigned dermatosis.[7] Where trauma is involved, the resultant wound often serves

Table 12-2. Features Suggestive of Factitial Skin Disease

1. Morphology unlike any known genuine dermatosis.
   —geometric lesions
   —linear lesions
   —lesions distributed in accessible sites
2. Lesions appear in fully developed form, usually at night.
3. Secondary gain a factor monetary or emotional.
4. A real lesion often precedes the factitious eruption, occasionally providing a pattern.
5. The pattern is suggestive factitious until proven otherwise.
   —cutaneous gangrene
   —extremity edema with sharp margins
   —nonhealing surgical wounds
   —spontaneous symptomatic bruising
   —patients who bring containers of "bugs" into the office
6. Intolerance of dressings and bandages
7. Emotional immaturity

---

as the pattern for future factitial lesions.[8,9,10] In this case, unable to produce lesions remotely similar to leukocytoclastic vasculitis, Mr. W. resorted to the use of ligatures to produce swollen extremities. As in virtually all cases of factitial dermatoses, the pattern produced is unlike any known genuine cutaneous abnormality, and yet he successfully fooled numerous physicians for many years.

A pivotal question then is how could he succeed with what is a rather obvious hoax? First, let me say that this case is by no means unusual or more obvious than most.[11,12,13] A supporting medical history, , of an unusual and poorly defined medical syndrome (the brief episode of vasculitis in this case), surely clouded the consciousness of subsequent examiners. It is difficult to see the self-induced nature of the process (the forest) in light of previous notes, biopsy reports, etc., regarding "leukocytoclastic vasculitis" (the trees). To avoid this pitfall, our initial visual impressions should be virgin, untainted by historical information. It is far easier to have a second look, after absorbing historical information, than to remove the influence of such information on our perceptions.

Key elements in the evaluation of Mr. W. are pertinent to all three types of factitial disease (Table 12-3). Photography is crucial for documentation and, on occasion, diagnosis. In fact, a clear appreciation of the pattern, and a clue to the means employed has, on occasion, emerged only on review of such photographic evidence. Plying the physician with details of past medical history, these patients are often skilled at concealing the true cause of their lesions at the bedside. A standard photographic approach is recommended. Full body overviews front and rear (to reveal the distribution), and close-ups of individual lesions (to help discriminate genuine from phony and perhaps suggest the means employed) are advised in every unusual chronic dermatosis. Such pictures are equally helpful in the diagnosis of genuine disease.

The diagnosis, even if obvious, may be confirmed by interfering in the traumatic manipulations of the patient. In this case, a full arm cast rapidly relieved the swelling by preventing place-

---

Table 12-3. Evaluation of Factitial Dermatoses

---

1. Virgin examination
2. Complete history
3. Total body photography, overviews, and close-ups
4. Protective bandaging
5. Biopsy of lesion (polarize, electron probe analysis)[a]
6. Microscopic analysis of nail scrapings[b]
7. Surprise visits
8. Search of patients' belongings[c,*]
9. One-way mirror[d,*]

---

[a]Jackson RM, Tucker SB, Abraham JL, Millns JL: Factitial cutaneous ulcers and nodules: The use of electron-probe microanalysis in diagnosis. *J Am Acad Derm* 1984; 11:1065–1069.
[b]Shelley WB: Factitial dermatitis as the presenting sign of multiple lentigines syndrome. *Arch Derm* 1982; 118:260–262.
[c]Lyell A: Cutaneous artifactual disease. *J Am Acad Derm* 1979; 1:391–407.
[d]White JG, Pearson HA, Coddington RD: Purpura factitia. *Clin Peds* 1966; 5:157–160.
*Felt to be illegal by one of our hospital attorneys.

ment of the ligatures. Be aware that, on occasion, such an approach will be furiously resisted with complaints of exquisite intolerance of even the most trifling of bandages. I have also been impressed with efforts by some patients to work around or even through the sturdiest of devices. Wounds so produced are rather obvious.

Additional studies may provide further proof of a factitious process but are unnecessary. For instance, previous authors have demonstrated blown-out lymphatics with lymphangiography and even grooving of the underlying bone on radiographic examination.[11,13] Additional study is better directed at ruling out a genuine underlying illness. One must always remember that malingerers are also susceptible to myocardial infarction, appendicitis, carcinoma, and other ailments. Unlike the fable, I assure you both the physician as well as the patient stand to suffer for failing to heed the cry of "wolf!"

Malingerers, when deeper psychosis is not suggested, may be safely confronted. The majority of patients will cooperate once found out. This group is by far the easiest to manage. Where insurance fraud, litigation, or unusual compensations are involved, careful documentation (especially photography) is crucial.

Case Number 2: Self-Mutilating Factitial Dermatosis

Ms. S., a twenty-seven year-old nursing administrator, was referred for evaluation of chronic nonhealing ulcerative skin lesions. Multiple biopsies demonstrated intense acute inflammation and ulceration of the epidermis and dermis with extension into subcutaneous fat. There was no evidence of vasculitis or systemic fungal infection. An extensive evaluation revealed no evidence for an underlying illness. Based on a diagnosis of pyoderma gangrenosum, multiple therapies were prescribed with limited success. Older lesions healed eventually with scarring and new lesions continued to appear in crops. Often Ms. S. was aware of a vague sensation where a lesion would later appear. She had endured this dermatosis for over a year prior to her referral and the only apparent gain was the sympathy and admiration of her colleagues and family for being able to carry on with such a burden. She continued to work most of this time except for several absences imposed by the physicians where she worked in the belief that her festering sores were a risk to patients. For this reason she was eventually moved from patient care to a desk job—a move she regretted deeply.

Her medical center evaluation was exhaustive and similarly nonenlightening. In fact, in retrospect, the more vigorously one pursued the workup, the more frequent was the appearance of new lesions. Ulcers, blisters, and hemorrhagic papules appeared most evenings. Islands of normal skin separating two lesions would vanish overnight. Numerous bacteria were present in all of these wounds and treatment with parenteral antibiotics continued throughout the hospitalization. The wounds themselves were surprisingly asymptomatic though even the slightest of bandages resulted in bitter complaining and were always removed by Ms. S. Entire excisional biopsy of a breast ulcer added no new information though it is noteworthy that Ms. S. removed her own sutures from the wound on the second post-op day. The biopsy site became a nonhealing sore.

Ms. S. was overweight and physically unattractive. Covered by weeping sores at the height of the process, she was in fact pitiful to behold. She confided to one of us a lifetime of unhappiness. She had been given up for adoption by her mother, a prostitute, who later returned to embarrass and ridicule her. Shortly before the onset of her "illness" she was allegedly sexually assaulted by a motorcycle gang one evening after work. She had not been able to discuss this with her husband, with whom she endured an unfulfilling marriage. Mr. S. was rarely seen during her multiple lengthy admissions. Ms. S. usually brought herself to the hospital unannounced, calling in distress from pay phones at local shopping malls.

Released from the hospital to pursue a series of therapeutic trials, she was eventually readmitted due to lack of a response. Cavitary lung lesions were noted on routine chest X ray and subsequent CT scanning. One of these was removed at open lung biopsy and the unusual histologic pattern was felt to be consistent with bronchocentric granulomatosis. During this admission, multiple photographs as suggested above were obtained and the indication of self-induced disease was convincing. All of the cutaneous lesions were in easily reachable parts of the skin. Furthermore, early lesions were uncannily similar in morphology and were always paired, suggesting an "outside job." A brief search of the patient's room while she was busy in the X-ray department disclosed a stunning array of surgical instruments.

The patient was confronted and she promptly left the hospital, hotly denying any role in her illness. The referring physician, having known the patient and her family for some time, was unable to accept that Ms. S. could mutilate herself in such a fashion, particularly in the absence of significant rewards. She was lost to follow-up. Eventually we learned she presented to another medical center where after a similar workup, identical conclusions were reached.

This case illustrates self-mutilators, the most serious factitial dermatosis, and also illustrates several key mistakes in patient management. To an outsider, the gains received are trivial compared to the destruction produced, and for this reason I do not consider this a case of simple malingering.[14] The pity and admiration of colleagues and supporters certainly boosted her self-image and perhaps explains her strange behavior. The reasons for the often complex behavior of these patients are often difficult to determine. A sparse literature discusses theoretical and enigmatic motives for the complex behavior of self-mutilators. In one particularly well-studied case, at least six separate motives were felt to be at play: 1) satisfaction for succeeding at the deception, 2) sexual gratification from general anesthesia, 3) the warmth of the doctor-patient relationship, 4) excitement from undergoing diagnostic procedures, 5) drug addiction, and 6) room and board.[4] This patient was asked why he endured agony for such apparently trivial rewards. He replied, "Pain can't be remembered, but pleasure can."[4] Never be misled that a process is too horrible to be self-induced. The most unimaginable horrors are often self-inflicted. I have seen a patient remove his thumb to obtain compensation. Limb amputation, bilateral enucleation, and even autocastration have been reported.[15,16] Slicing off part of his ear, Vincent van Gogh became both the most famous and the most analyzed of self-mutilators. That a recent discussion of van Gogh's motives covers over 30 pages underscores the complexity of such behaviors.[17] That van Gogh committed suicide 2 years thereafter emphasizes the potential gravity of self-mutilation.

Whatever the reason(s), one can assume there is both a motive and a reward. In time, as physicians, we would like to understand the reasons behind such unusual behavior. Though such an understanding would be helpful, it is not essential to good treatment. Our therapeutic goals remain the same in either case: symptomatic relief, prevention of further harm by the patient or the medical system, careful follow-up, keeping an open mind about the diagnosis, and treatment of complications of self-mutilation, such as infection. A terrible mistake is to label factitial what is not. A cardinal rule in dealing with these patients is to exclude serious underlying disease.

Consider the mistakes in the case of Ms. S. The diagnosis of factitial dermatosis should have been entertained at the outset in view of the bizarre appearance of the lesions, which were unlike any known dermatosis.[10,18] According to Stokes, gangrene is such an uncommon intrinsic disease of skin that the question of external causes must always be considered.[10] Intolerance of bandages and clear-cut evidence of tampering (suture removal) were further important clues (Table 12-2). Failing to recognize the nature of the process early resulted in an enormously expensive and potentially hazardous investigation. It became clear that the harder we pushed to make a diagnosis, the more elaborate and mutilating the process became. In a case reported by Thomas, failure to make the correct diagnosis resulted in 33 stepwise amputations of one arm.[19] The economic cost of factitial illness can be awesome, and is certainly one reason to avoid exhaustive investigation in the absence of solid indications. A striking example is the case referenced by Scoggin in which the medical indebtedness reached $7 million.[5] We spent in excess of $30 thousand in the case of Ms. S., worsening considerably her financial well-being.

The appropriate response in such cases is to let the patient know that they have found someone to care for them and look after them: "Though I cannot fully explain your problem, I have had experience with similar cases and will be happy to look after you. I will see you as often as needed at your convenience." According to Lyell, the situation is likened to dealing with terrorists holding hostages where the essence is to maintain contact.[7] Frequent visits are far cheaper than frequent tests. When caring for such patients our goal is always to avoid adding to their suffering with therapeutic misadventures and costly medical bills. Building a close relationship with the patient is more apt to be beneficial than unnecessary, expensive, and often hazardous diagnostic testing. I discourage potentially hazardous treatment and in some cases find placebo therapy very useful.

The natural history of self-mutilation is unknown. The role of psychotherapy is also uncertain since in most cases psychotherapy is refused.[20] In one retrospective series of 43 patients, 33 were available for follow-up. Of these, 20 were known to have resolved their factitious eruptions and 13 continued to produce lesions a mean of 12.4 years later.[20] Self-mutilation implies a serious personality disturbance or psychosis.[21] Ms. S. had been interviewed by our psychiatry service but was uncooperative. She refused further discussion with our psychiatric consultant but agreed to begin a trial of antidepressant medication which was singularly unsuccessful and, according to her, "not worth the side effects." The problem returns to the domain of the primary physician or dermatologic consultant.

Direct confrontation is inadvisable in light of the serious psychopathology associated with surreptitious self-mutilation. While one may be successful with such a direct approach, dire consequences have resulted in up to a third of such patients in some series.[11] So far this has not happened to Ms. S. Stripped of an albeit abnormal coping mechanism and threatened with the discovery by their friends and loved ones, attempted suicide is often a substitute response. In situations where one is of the opinion that immediate confrontation is required for the safety of the patient, it should be made clear to the patient that the true nature of the process will be kept in confidence. In such situations, seasoned dermatologists advise that one infers knowledge of what is going on rather than pointing the finger with accusation.[10,22] One should never enlist the family in a plot against the patient, nor tell the family what is going on. There is bound to be a great deal of resentment that may surface, to the detriment of the patient at a time when support is badly needed. There is nothing to be served by bringing the wrath of what few supporters are available on such a fragile person. Furthermore, confrontation often invites wrath upon the physician. "It is disconcerting at times, after one's efforts to establish a proved case to find the family physician unconvinced because he cannot reconcile the diagnosis with his own opinion of the patient's integrity and moral caliber."[10]

Case Number 3: Pickers and Scratchers

"It is better than riches to scratch where it itches."[23]

Mr. and Mrs. G. presented to the clinic with numerous excoriated papules covering all parts of the body accessible to scratching. He complained bitterly of itching. His symptoms had been present for 2 years and exhaustive physical and laboratory examination had not revealed any abnormality. Mr. and Mrs. G.'s house had been exterminated on several occasions. The patient was convinced that he was infested with insects and brought samples of these "bugs" for us to examine. Mr. G. also brought a tube of toothpaste and other household products he thought were infested. In the last year his wife had become similarly "infested." Desperate, the couple sprayed themselves and all their personal belongings with potent insecticides and moved from Florida to North Carolina to escape the infestation. They continued to suffer and sought advice from a local physician. Despite his best efforts at symptomatic therapy with topical and systemic steroids and multiple antihistamines, the couple had little relief.

Physical examination was remarkable only for the self-inflicted lesions. Laboratory studies were normal. The samples he produced were not insects but bits of epidermal and dermal debris. Using his comb, Mr. G. demonstrated that the material moved, apparently due to static electricity. Freshly plucked bits of dermis will also appear to move due to elasticity of the tissue, often convincing the plucker there is something crawling under their skin.

The couple was unsatisfied by our analysis but agreed to try a therapy we mentioned might help the situation. They were persuaded to discontinue topical insecticides and were given bland emollients instead. The antipsychotic medication haloperidol was begun at a dose of 1 mg twice daily and promptly relieved symptoms in both patients.

This group includes a variety of self-inflicted dermatoses that share common features (Table 1). Patients in this group readily admit that they are injuring their skin and in time the picking and scratching becomes habitual. Often, as in other factitious eruptions, a genuine dermatosis precedes the factitious or habitual condition. For example, a patient infested with scabies may scratch habitually months and years after they are cleared of scabies mites. Such patients are commonly said to have neurodermatitis. The latter term has no place in medical jargon. Such a diagnosis is very distasteful to patients and conveys little information. Historically, even such well accepted skin disorders as atopic dermatitis were once regarded as disseminated neurodermatitis.[24] It is a travesty to label sufferers as neurotic. According to Sulzberger, "one need have no further therapeutic failures" if everything unexplained is neurotic or psychosomatic in origin.[25] In this group especially, one must keep an open mind about the diagnosis. Pruritus is a common symptom of systemic disease.[26]

The underlying motives in the case of Mr. and Mrs. G were never appreciated. Several authors have ascribed delusional parasitosis to repressed sexuality, guilt, or anger, but have mixed feelings about the value of psychiatric referral.[17,27,28] Our approach is first to exclude a real infestation. Contrary to popular opinion, some of the "bugs" brought in by patients really are insects. Therefore, all such samples must be examined. The home may need to be inspected, since many biting insects do not live on their victim, would not be seen in the doctor's office, and would not be affected by topical insecticides such as lindane (Kwell). Having done our best to eliminate the possibility of a genuine infestation or metabolic cause of pruritus, a trial of low dose haloperidol is prescribed along with soothing topical emollients. In many cases this approach is successful. Psychiatric referral is reserved for those patients who fail to respond.

Most pickers and scratchers do not have delusions of parisitosis. They simply itch, or rather feel an urge to scratch. For the majority of such patients, no explanation for their symptoms will be found on investigation, though investigation of persistent pruritus is always a good idea.[26] I have seen several patients carrying the diagnosis of neurodermatitis who proved to have lymphoma, iron deficiency anemia, sclerosing cholangitis, and the like. Often the underlying diagnosis remains obscure for years, suggesting a need for long-term follow-up. A label of neurodermatitis tends to close the door on objective thinking and leaves the patient with the notion they are somehow neurotic. Such a patient who was subsequently found to have Hodgkin's disease exclaimed a sigh of relief, "At least I'm not crazy!" In the absence of a remedial diagnosis, empiric therapy with antihistamines is suggested. A favorite soothing topical preparation for generalized pruritus of any cause is limewater/olive oil emulsion with 1 percent camphor and ½ percent phenol added.

There are those who habitually scratch without itching, bite their nails, or pluck hair. Mildly disfiguring, these habits are really not as serious as cigarette smoking. Rarely do these conditions indicate serious emotional disturbances, though stress likely influences the behavior. Protecting patients from unconscious self-destruction usually extinguishes the habit. For instance, those who pluck their hair (trichotillo mania) are best treated with a hairpiece.

Intellectually and emotionally, patients with psychocutaneous syndromes are extraordinarily challenging. Many of the references present incredibly fascinating case histories.[2,6,7,10] Overall, the prognosis is excellent. The majority of therapeutic failures are attributable to physician error. Pitfalls abound. Mistakes are made both in failing to exclude genuine illness and overspending to do so. A high index of suspicion improves the chances for accurate diagnosis. Psychiatric referral is rarely necessary and often unsuccessful. The best doctor to manage the patient is the first doctor who recognizes the problem. Successful therapy requires only the ability to recognize those patients with serious emotional disturbances and the willingness to provide safe, compassionate, long-term care.

REFERENCES

1. Shelley WB: Dermatitis artefacta induced in a patient by one of her multiple personalities. *Br J Derm* 1981; 105:587–589.
2. Ormsby OS: Factitious dermatoses. *JAMA* 1915; 65:1622–1628.

3. Reich P, Gottfried LA: Factitious disorders in a teaching hospital. *Ann Intern Med* 1983; 99:240–247.
4. Justus PG, Kreutzioer SS, Kitchens CS: Probing the dynamics of Munchausen's syndrome. *Ann Intern Med* 1980; 93:120–127.
5. Scoggin CH: Factitious illness: Dramatic deceit versus reality. *Postgrad Med* 1983; 74:259–265.
6. Hawkings JR, Jones KS, Sim M, Tibbetts RW: Deliberate disability. *Br Med J* 1956; 1:361–367.
7. Lyell A: Cutaneous artifactual disease. *J Am Acad Derm* 1979; 1:391–407.
8. Gandy DT: The concept and clinical aspects of factitial dermatitis. *Southern Med J* 1953; 46:551–555.
9. Lancashire GH: Dermatitis artefacta. *Br Med J* 1922; 2:504–505.
10. Stokes JH, Garner VC: The diagnosis of self inflicted lesions of the skin. *JAMA* 1929; 93:438–443.
11. Smith RJ: Factitious lymphedema of the hand. *J Bone and Joint Surg* 1975; 57:89–94.
12. Knight A, James PS: Elastic band artifact. *Proc Roy Soc Med* 1976; 69:383–384.
13. Kitchin ID, McGibbon C, Seville RH: Artifact ulcers and bone lesions produced by elastic bands. *Br Med J* 1967; 2:218–219.
14. Hollender MH, Abram HS: Dermatitis factitia. *South Med J* 1973; 66:1279–1285.
15. Gorin M: Self-inflicted bilateral enucleation. *Arch Ophthalmology* 1964; 72:225–226.
16. Kushner AW: Two cases of auto castration due to relibious delusions. *Br J Med Psychol* 1967; 40:293–298.
17. Lubin AJ: Vincent van Gogh's ear. *Psychoanal Q* 1961; 30:351–384.
18. Waisman M: Pickers, pluckers and impostors: A panorama of cutaneous self-mutilation. *Postgrad Med J* 1965; 38:620–630.
19. Thomas EWP. Dermatitis artefacta: A note on an unusual case. *Br Med J* 1937; 1:804–806.
20. Sneddon I, Sneddon J: Self-inflicted injury: A follow-up study of 43 patients. *Br Med J* 1975; 3:527–530.

21. Koblenzer CS: Psychosomatic concepts in dermatology. *Arch Derm* 1983; 119:501–511.
22. Callaway JL: Personal communication, 1982.
23. Anonymous.
24. Lynch FW, Hinkley RG, Cowan DW: Psychosomatic studies in dermatology. Disseminate neurodermatitis. *Arch Derm Syph* 1945; 51:251–260.
25. Cornblect T, Brown M: Dermatologic manifestations in psychiatric disorders. *JAMA* 1948; 136:152–157.
26. Lyell A: The itching patient. *Scot Med J* 1972; 17:334–347.
27. Michelson HE: Psychosomatic studies in dermatology: The motivation of self-induced eruptions. *Arch Derm Syph* 1945; 51:245–250.
28. Jackson RM, Tucker SB, Abraham JL, Millins JL: Factitial cutaneous ulcers and nodules: The use of electron-probe microanalysis in diagnosis. *J Am Acad Derm* 1984; 11:1065–1069.

Chapter 13

FACTITIAL FEVER

Harry A. Gallis, M.D.

Introduction

Fever is a common symptom or finding in medical practice. Patients frequently complain of feeling feverish with chills or sweats. Many of these episodes are acute febrile illnesses which are self-limited, resolve without therapy, and usually represent common viral infections. Clinical judgment and careful physical examination usually separate benign and potentially serious problems. This chapter will concentrate on individuals who have the findings of or complain of prolonged fever in whom no etiology is readily apparent and in whom there is reason to suspect psychiatric or self-induced illness.

Much has been written on the subject of fever of unknown origin (FUO) and it is beyond the scope of this chapter to discuss it in great detail. However, for the purposes of definition, it is essential to review differential diagnoses. Fever of unknown origin, as described in the classic article of Petersdorf and Beeson[1] refers to illnesses of 3 weeks in duration with fever higher than 101° F or 38.3°C in whom no diagnosis is made during 1 week's investigation in hospital. The most common groups of diseases encountered in these patients are infectious (e.g. intra-abdominal abscess, mycobacterial infection, urinary tract infection, etc.), malignant (especially lymphomas, leukemias, and intra-abdominal solid tumors), and collagen vascular (vasculitis, systemic lupus erythematosus, inflammatory arthropathies, etc.). These three categories account for approximately 80 percent of the patients in most studies. Five to 15 percent are undiagnosed and usually resolve; however, 3 to 5 percent are found to be factitious or self-induced.

Another group of patients who generally do not meet the criteria for selection in these reviews (because of low-grade fever) are equally perplexing and have been referred to in the literature as periodic fever, psychogenic fever, or hysterical hyperthermia. These patients are usually younger and have symptoms out of proportion to physical and laboratory findings. The remainder of this discussion will deal with the diagnostic and therapeutic approaches to these patients and patients with factitious or self-induced illness.

CLINICAL EVALUATION

Regardless of the severity of illness, a systematic evaluation must be initiated on each patient. If the patient has not been previously examined by other physicians, inpatient or outpatient evaluation is begun. A thorough medical history includes careful inquiry into prescription and over-the-counter drug use, travel, animal exposures, occupational exposures, exposure to individuals with infectious illness, as well as the fever pattern. Written documentation of fever cannot be overemphasized. In this initial interview the physician begins to examine the patient's response to illness. A thorough and complete physical evaluation follows. If the individual appears acutely ill, hospitalization is warranted. On the other hand, if the patient appears well or there is insufficient documentation of fever, the patient should be asked to measure his temperature orally and record the values, times, and dates. Careful instruction should be given to avoid taking the temperature immediately after ingestion of hot or cold foods or liquids or after smoking.

Initial laboratory examination should include a complete blood count, urinalysis, erythrocyte sedimentation rate (ESR), blood chemistries (especially liver function tests), chest roentgenogram, cultures of appropriate body fluids, and any serologic or other blood tests indicated by the history and physical.

If fever is not documented (i.e., maximal daily temperatures 99.5°F) the patient should be reassured and followed. If fever is documented or the patient is vague and noncompliant in temperature taking (but usually complaining of various problems) hospitalization is warranted for documentation of abnormal temperature initially using oral temperatures. In most hospitals, temperatures are now taken with electronic thermometers under direct supervision of nursing personnel. If this is not the case, one must be aware of the potential for manipulation (hot liquids, friction, etc.) of glass thermometers or actual swapping of thermometers with preset temperatures. Checking serial numbers will be useful if this is suspected. In a review of factitious fever and self-induced infection, Aduan et al.[2] suspected or documented thermometer manipulation of 19 of 32 patients while self-induced infections were seen in 13 others.

FACTITIOUS OR SELF-INDUCED ILLNESS

Patients with these presentations are frequently perplexing to the primary care physician. The presenting symptoms and signs are usually dramatic or documented. It generally takes a certain degree of familiarity with a patient before one begins to suspect a manipulative personality. In the series of patients with factitious illness reviewed by Aduan[2] 20 of 32 patients were referred with FUO, 10 with recurrent skin infections with or without bacteremia, and one each with systemic vasculitis and abdominal granulomata, respectively. Only 4 of 32 had been documented to have psychiatric illness and only 10 of 32 were suspected of factitious illness prior to referral. These 32 patients accounted for 10 percent of the patients referred to the National Institutes of Health for an FUO protocol.

In the group of patients found to have factitious fever, 19 were manipulating thermometers by application of heat or friction or shaking the thermometers in the reverse direction. The signs leading to the proper diagnosis of these patients are outlined in Table 13-1. In general, if factitious illness is suspected, the patient should be allowed to "perform" so that the diagnosis may be solidly established. Once an unusual or suspicious fever pattern is observed, supervised oral and rectal temperatures should be taken. Others have recommended taking the temperature of freshly voided urine, which correlates well with rectal temperatures. These temperatures should be normal in patients who manipulate thermometers.

Another subgroup of patients induces true infection and fever by self-inoculation with infectious or pyrogenic materials. Injection with feces, bacterial cultures, milk, and tetanus toxid have all been documented in the literature.[2] Injection sites are usually anatomically distributed over accessible body areas, e.g., anterior thighs and abdomen rather than back or buttocks. These patients, of course, have true fever and may have associated single

Table 13-1. Signs in the Diagnosis of Factitious Fever*

1. Fever without evidence of active disease at physical examination or on screening diagnostic tests.
2. Absence of tachycardia with abrupt temperature spikes.
3. Discrepancy between patient's physical examination findings and apparent very high temperature, particularly the absence of skin warmth.
4. Apparent rapid defervescence (within minutes), unaccompanied by diaphoresis.
5. Marked hyperpyrexia 41.1°C.
6. Lack of diurnal variation in temperature, reversal of diurnal variation, or other unusual temperature pattern.
7. Marked discrepancy between oral and rectal temperatures taken simultaneously.
8. No fever with nurse or physical attending.
9. Other associated factitious disease.

*Tables 13-1, 13-2, and 13-3 are from Aduan RP, Fauci AS, Dale CD, Herzberg JH, Wolff SM: Factitious fever and self-induced infection. *Ann Int Med* 1979; 90:230–242.

organism or polymicrobial bacteremias. The majority of these patients are medical personnel.

Underlying Psychiatric Illnesses

The management of patients with FUO frequently necessitates psychiatric consultation. In patients in whom organic illness is suspected or documented, management of anxiety and depression is frequently necessary. In addition, in situations of excessive somatization or factitious illness, psychiatric evaluation should be presented to the patient as being a part of the routine evaluation of all such patients, and, if necessary, to evaluate how "the stress of the illness" is affecting the patient's current condition. The attending physician should discuss the patient with the psychiatrist prior to consultation.

The most common psychiatric diagnosis in patients with factitious illness is that of "borderline personality disorder" (Table 13-2) characterized by impulsive and manipulative behavior, poor reality testing, defects in self-esteem, concealed anger and hostility, and episodic self-destructive acting out.[2,3,4,5] Another large group are experiencing conversion reactions, and organic illnesses must be carefully excluded. Patients with depression, anxiety, and adjustment reactions may be encountered, as well as individuals in whom secondary gain is involved (lawsuits, disability, or other compensation) (Table 13-3).

Management

Once psychiatric evaluation has been completed, the physicians and other ward personnel should meet to discuss the findings and plan strategy. This conference should include the patient's attending physician, psychiatrist, psychologist, social worker, nursing staff, and family members as indicated. The documentation of factitious illness or thermometer manipulation should be assembled. If sufficient data are lacking and the patient's illness is life threatening, room searches for needles, syringes, extra thermometers, etc. may be necessary. When all data and assessments are assembled, the patient may be confronted in a nonaccusational and nonpunitive manner. Hostility and an-

Table 13-2. Characteristics of Patients with Borderline Syndrome

1. Identity disturbance
    a. Lack of a coherent self-identity (identity diffusion)
    b. Uncertainty about self-image, gender identity, long-term goals
2. Intense affect
    a. Acts in an angry and negativistic way
    b. Depression—existential despair
3. Inadequate impulse control
    a. Episodic self-destructive acts; intent is not self-harm or self-punishment, but rather object manipulation or establishment of self-identity.
4. Deficient sense of reality
    a. Imperfect discrimination/differentiation between self and significant objects
    b. Disturbed states of consciousness—inability to distinguish between dreaming an experience and reality (depersonalization, dissociation, derealization)
5. Brief psychotic episodes
    a. Psychotic symptoms (regression) usually precipitated by life stress or transference in psychotherapy
6. Unstable interpersonal relations
    a. Constantly using others for own needs
    b. Everyday relationships superficial and transient
    c. Close relationships, when existent, are intense, with demanding, manipulative, clinging, dependent behavior.
    d. Use of rapid superficial identification with others (mimicry)
7. Adequate social functioning
    a. Behaves appropriately and adaptively
    b. Has problems tolerating being alone and thus tends not to be socially withdrawn.
    c. General lack of creative achievement over time

ger are usually directed toward the physicians and hence, it is valuable to perform this maneuver in a ward setting in which nursing and other personnel are psychiatrically trained so that they may begin supportive care. Provisions must be made for initial inpatient therapy with adequate psychiatric follow-up after

Table 13-3. Guidelines for Management of Patients with Borderline Syndrome

1. Early psychiatric consultation is imperative for the staff to understand the complexities of the patient's behavior and their role in his illness.
2. Reestablishment of open staff communication to prevent staff splitting and inconsistencies in the patient's day-to-day management.
3. Acknowledgment of the "real" stresses in the patient's situation and their relation to the patient's sense of entitlement.
4. Recognizing the primitive defense mechanisms of the patient (splitting, primitive idealization, projective identification, feeling of omnipotence, and devaluation).
5. Empathic limit-setting, without punishment or rejection.
6. Anticipation of repeated unrealistic expectations, and regressive self-destructive acting-out after disappointment.

discharge. For further reading in this area, the reader is referred to guidelines in the management of borderline patients.[2,7]

LOW GRADE FEVER AND EXCESSIVE CONCERN

Fortunately, true factitious illness remains an uncommon problem. More frequently, the physician encounters the patient who is experiencing "recurrent infections," "sore throat," or "low-grade fever." These patients frequently give a history of an antecedent acute febrile illness, often diagnosed on clinical grounds as infectious mononucleosis, and usually complain of temperatures of 99–100° F, sweats, fatigue, poor sleep habits, weight gain or loss, and recurrent sore throat or swollen cervical lymph nodes. There is a significant subgroup of these individuals who have normal temperatures and claim that their "normal" temperature is "sub normal." Physical and laboratory evaluations are infrequently rewarding and significant diagnosable illnesses rarely develop. In the NIH series reported by Aduan[5], psychiatric diagnoses were more common in this group of patients than in those in whom an etiology for FUO was determined. It should be noted that these patients, on hospitalization, do not meet the artificial criteria established for FUO (temp. ⩾ 101.5°) and perhaps should be dubbed "FUO minor." Much attention has been drawn to the syndrome of chronic mononucleosis, which includes the subgroup of these patients who have persistent high titer Epstein Barr viral capsid antigen (⩾ 1:320) and early antigen (⩾ 1:10) antibodies. This is thought to represent a state of abnormal handling of Epstein Barr virus with presumed ongoing infection causing persistence of the fatigue seen in acute infectious mononucleosis. It should be noted, however, that Henle et al.[8] have reviewed the serologic data on a large group of mononucleosis patients and cannot distinguish serologically those who recovered and those who had persistent symptoms. The approach to these patients is similar to that of other somatization disorders, with psychiatric consultation and therapy where indicated, and careful routine follow-up with reassurance. It is possible that the mild temperature elevation seen in some of these patients is only an exaggeration of normal brought to light by temperature taking during an acute symptomatic illness. Many individuals are not aware of the normal diurnal variation of body temperature and it is helpful to point this out in a reassuring manner. It should be noted that hemoglobin, ESR, and serum albumin are usually normal in this group of patients.

The prognosis is variable and depends on the duration of symptoms and underlying psychiatric diagnoses. Evolution into illnesses seen in standard FUO series is unusual. Most patients improve with time but may not feel normal for several years. The true role of "mononucleosis agents" (EBV, cytomegalovirus, and toxoplasma) is unclear.

References

1. Petersdorf RG, Beeson PB: Fever of unexplained origin: Report on 100 cases. *Med* 1961; 40:1–30.
2. Aduan RP, Fauci AS, Dale CD, Herzberg JH, Wolff SM: Factitious fever and self-induced infection. *Ann Int Med* 1979; 90:230–242.

3. Groves JE: Management of the borderline patient on a medical or surgical ward: The psychiatric consultant's role. *Int J Psychiatry Med* 1975; 6:337–348.
4. Groves JE: Borderline personality disorder. *N Engl J Med* 1981; 305:259–262.
5. Aduan RP: Psychiatric aspects of FUO. In *FUO: Fever of Undetermined Origin*. Mount Kisco, NY, 1983 Futura, pp. 321–340.
6. Adler G: Hospital treatment of borderline patients. *Am J Psychiatry* 1973; 130:32–36.
7. Groves JE: Taking care of the hateful patient. *N Engl J Med* 1978; 298:883–887.
8. Henle W *et al:* Long-term serological follow-up of patients for Epstein-Barr virus after recovery from infectious mononucleosis. *J Infec Dis* 1985; 151:1150–1153.

Part V

PSYCHSOMATIC MEDICINE REVISITED

Chapter 14

EXCESSIVE SOMATIC CONCERN

Diagnostic and Treatment Issues

J. Trig Brown, M.D.
John I. Walker, M.D.

In certain clinical situations, either no organic explanation can be found for a patient's complaints, or the complaints seem disproportionate to the severity of the physical findings. This phenomenon we call "excessive somatic concern" and it includes several diagnostic categories (Table 14-1) which will be reviewed. Characteristics of the different clinical syndromes will be highlighted, and guidelines will be offered for managing these complicated patients.

SYMPTOM FORMATION

The diagnostician would be out of work if every symptom was easily reduced to its cause. Figure 14-1 schematically represents factors which can effect symptom formation. In the upper half of Figure 14-1, the artificial one-to-one relationship between a peripheral sensation and symptom production is represented. In clinical medicine, this straight-forward representation is the exception rather than the rule. No two patients with similar pathophysiological problems have identical symptoms. The mul-

Table 14-1. Excessive Somatic Concern

Somatoform Disorders
Factitious Illnesses
Depression
Grief Reactions
Anxiety
Organic Brain Syndromes
Psychoses

tiple factors related to symptoms variability are depicted by the bottom half of Figure 14-1. The brain is that area where the peripheral sensations are processed prior to symptom formation, and no two patients have identical symptoms because of the variability of individuals' brains. The brain's activity could result in the sensation being minimized and no symptoms produced (this phenomenon may explain noncompliant patients, denying patients, etc); or, as described in detail in this chapter, amplified. This central amplification process can be viewed as the primary problem in patients with excessive somatic concern. Several factors influence the individual's susceptibility or resistance to symptom formation. Genetic defects may predispose the individual to certain patterns of symptom formation. Innate differences in sensitivity and temperament and activity level produce varied responses to environmental pressures. Childhood emo-

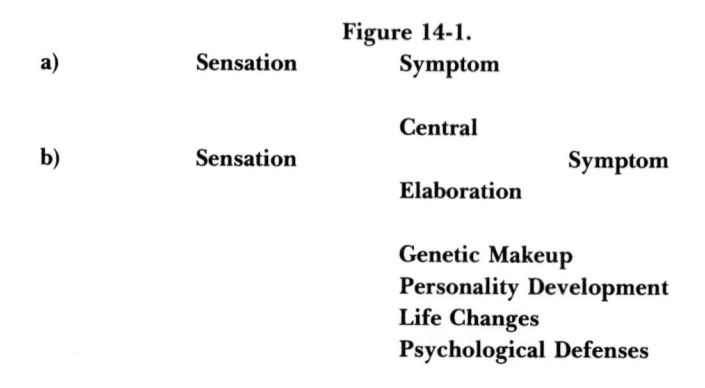

Figure 14-1.

a) Sensation → Symptom

b) Sensation → Central Elaboration → Symptom

Genetic Makeup
Personality Development
Life Changes
Psychological Defenses

tional trauma, such as maternal deprivation during the infant stage of development, may induce the greater sensitivity to environmental stress in adulthood. Parental rejection, overprotection, and overpermissiveness result in increased vulnerability to environmental pressures. Undesirable parental models, early communication failures, sibling rivalry, poverty, and low economic status may interfere with a mature response to stress.

In the late 1960s, Holmes and Rahe devised the social readjustment rating scale (Table 14-2) ranking the environmental

Table 14-2. The Social Readjustment Rating Scale*

Life Event	Life Change Units
1. Death of spouse	100
2. Divorce	73
3. Marital separation	65
4. Jail term	63
5. Death of a close family member	63
6. Personal injury or illness	53
7. Marriage	50
8. Fired at work	47
9. Marital reconciliation	45
10. Retirement	45
11. Change in health of family member	44
12. Pregnancy	40
13. Sex difficulties	39
14. Gain of new family member	39
15. Business readjustment	39
16. Change in financial state	38
17. Death of a close friend	37
18. Change to different line of work	36
19. Change in number of arguments with spouse	35
20. Mortgage over $10,000	31
21. Foreclosure of mortgage or loan	30
22. Change in responsibilities at work	29
23. Son or daughter leaving home	29
24. Trouble with in-laws	29
25. Outstanding personal achievement	28

Table 14-2. The Social Readjustment Rating Scale*
(continued)

26. Wife beginning or stopping work	26
27. Beginning or ending school	26
28. Change in living conditions	25
29. Revision of personal habits	24
30. Trouble with boss	23
31. Change in work hours or conditions	20
32. Change in residence	20
33. Change in schools	20
34. Change in recreation	19
35. Change in church activities	19
36. Change in social activities	18
37. Mortgage or loan less than $10,000	17
38. Change in sleeping habits	16
39. Change in number of family get-togethers	15
40. Change in eating habits	15
41. Vacation	13
42. Christmas	12
43. Minor violations of the law	11

*From Holmes TH, Rahe RH: The Social Readjustment Rating Scale. *J Psychosom Res* 1967; 11:213.

stresses that contribute to symptom formation. Their scale compares 43 life events according to the severity of their impact. Holmes and Rahe rate the death of a spouse as the most significant life event, giving this stress a value of 100 points, whereas a minor infraction of the law has the value of 11 points. Other life events include divorce, at 73 points; pregnancy, 40 points; and troubles with in-laws, 29 points. When events over a 12-month period total 150 to 199 points, approximately 25 percent of the population develop illness; with 200 to 299 points, 50 percent of the population become symptomatic; and with over 300 points, 79 percent of the population develop physical or emotional symptoms.

Psychological defense mechanisms effect symptom formation. Defense mechanisms are categorized into four types: primitive defense mechanisms, character defense mechanisms, neurotic defense mechanisms, and mature defense mechanisms. Individuals who consistently employ primitive defense mechanisms tend to decompensate under stress; individuals who use mature defense mechanisms tolerate high levels of stress.

Primitive defense mechanisms more commonly found in psychotic individuals include distortions (hallucinations and illusions), delusions (false beliefs), and oral fixations (helpless surrender and clinging behavior). These defense mechanisms result from psychodynamic conflicts occurring in the earliest stages of child development.

Character defense mechanisms include projection (the transference of an individual's unacceptable thoughts or feelings onto others), denial (the rejection of external reality), and passive-aggressive behavior (the indirect expression of hostility through procrastination, withholding, "innocent" mistakes, and other provocative behavior that is ultimately self-defeating).

Neurotic defense mechanisms, used by individuals who exhibit no gross distortion in reality testing or personality disorganization partially modify the individual's unconscious feelings and impulses. Neurotic defense mechanisms include repression (the unconscious exclusion of ideas or impulses from the individual's awareness), reaction formation (the development of feelings or ideas that are completely contrary to an individual's unconscious feelings or ideas), intellectualization (constant rumination over conflicts), regression (withdrawal to an earlier developmental level), and displacement (the redirection of feelings from an emotionally charged person or situation to a less threatening person or object).

Mature defense mechanisms are found in individuals who have stable marriages, good physical health, a rewarding career, and the ability to enjoy recreational activities. Mature defense mechanisms enable the individual to integrate unconscious sexual and aggressive drives with the demands of reality. These individuals are less critical and demanding of themselves and others. Mature defense mechanisms include altruism (constructive service to others), suppression (the conscious decision to delay paying attention to an uncomfortable impulse or conflict), anticipation (goal-directed planning for the future), and humor.

It is through better understanding of the interrelations of the multiple factors that affect the central elaboration process that one can better understand the patients with excessive somatic concern.

SOMATOFORM DISORDERS

The primary examples of excessive somatic concern occur in the somatoform disorders. An individual with a somatoform disorder has physical complaints with no demonstrable organic findings. The symptom of a patient with a somatoform disorder is linked to psychological conflict. Currently there are five varieties of the somatoform disorders (Table 14-3).

Somatization Disorder

The key to making the diagnosis of somatization disorder involves the polysymptomatic nature of the complaints and the facts that the patient has generally undergone many surgeries. These patients have multiple symptoms ranging from every organ system of the body (Table 14-4). The illness begins before the age of thirty and has a chronic course with some fluctuation. These patients are prone to numerous surgical procedures and tend to develop drug dependency. This disorder is seen predominantly in females, although not exclusively. About 1 percent of the general population has somatization disorder.

The typical patient with somatization disorder would be seen in the general medical clinic at about the age of thirty-five. Her

Table 14-3. Somatoform Disorders

Somatization disorder
Hypochondriasis
Conversion disorder
Psychogenic pain disorder
Atypical somatoform disorder

Table 14-4. Somatization-Polysymptomatic

sickly	seizures, paralysis
difficulty swallowing	trouble walking
loss of voice	dysuria
deafness	urinary retention
double/blurred vision	shortness of breath
blindness	palpitations
fainting, dizziness	chest pain
abdominal pain	menstrual irregularity
nausea	excessive bleeding
vomiting	vomiting in pregnancy
bloating	sexual indifference
food intolerance	lack of sexual pleasure
diarrhea	dyspareunia, genital pain
painful menstruation	back, joint pain

past medical history would be notable for an appendectomy at the age of fourteen, a right oophorectomy at the age of fifteen because of an ovarian cyst, a left oophorectomy at the age of seventeen because of a cyst, an ultimately a hysterectomy, cholecystectomy, and at least one exploratory laparotomy. The past medical history may also uncover a period of time with difficulty with "sick" (migraine-type) headaches that ultimately lead to narcotic dependence. Often the patient is seen in pain with a dramatic and seemingly exaggerated presentation.

Differential Diagnosis. Exaggerated physical complaints, the hallmark of a somatization disorder, can also be found in other conditions. Depressed patients may complain of fatigue, decreased appetite, diminished sexual interest, and constipation but, unlike the patient with a somatization disorder, disturbance in mood predominates and the illness presents acutely. Patients with somatization disorder may be chronically anxious, but their symptoms and course are usually different than those of generalized anxiety disorders. Patients with a conversion disorder or hypochondriasis do not demonstrate the multiple complaints found in a somatization disorder. Schizophrenic patients often have bizarre somatic delusions; patients with somatization disorder do not have delusions. Endocrine disorders, porphyria, multiple sclerosis, systemic lupus erythematosis, pernicious anemia, and other more common medical illnesses are characterized by multiple symptoms that may mimic a somatization disorder.

Psychodynamics. Somatization disorder can be explained as displacement of anxiety to the body. Often, patients with somatization disorders had inadequate relationships with others in their childhoods, generating considerable anxiety. These patients have learned to defend against this anxiety by gaining affection and care through illness.

Treatment. These patients are very difficult to treat. Ideally, understanding the dynamics of a patient's illness provides the key to treatment. Since patients with a somatization disorder seek a relationship of concern and care, placebos, reassurance, and psychiatric explanations fail to help them. Reassurance that nothing is physically wrong is viewed as a rejection, leading to an escalation of complaints. The indiscriminant use of placebos and other medication interferes with the development of a physician/patient relationship and produces an increase in complaints. Psychiatric explanations increase physical complaints.

When treating these patients, the physician must try to provide the patient with a stable and long-standing relationship. From the first interview, the physician should allow the patient some time to talk about the symptoms. Encouraging the patient to speak freely without interruption establishes a good physician/patient relationship and saves time and frustration in the long run by helping to prevent unnecessary telephone calls and visits in the middle of the night.

Unnecessary tests and treatments should be avoided after an initial diagnostic workup has been completed. Establishing a relationship with the patient offers the best treatment. The physician can offer support in the following manner:

> All the necessary diagnostic tests reveal nothing life threatening. Just because the tests demonstrated no source

for your symptoms does not mean that your symptoms are not significant. It is obvious that you are experiencing tremendous discomfort. Although I can't relieve all your symptoms, I would like to work with you to help you manage them more effectively.

Regular appointment times should be established with the patient and the patient should be encouraged to keep the appointment no matter how well he is feeling. This plan indicates that the physician cares for the patient, it diminishes complaints, and establishes a relationship based on trust rather than on illness. Initially, the patient may be seen for 30 minutes once or twice weekly. As a trusting relationship develops, the duration of a patient's visit can be diminished.

An increase in the patient's physical complaints often indicates environmental stresses. During this time, the physician should encourage more frequent appointments until the complaints have disappeared, thus preventing unnecessary diagnostic workups, medication, , and "physician-shopping." On the other hand, a change in the patient's physical complaints may indicate a new illness. Needless to say, Patients with somatization disorder can develop physical illness.

Patients often request medication. If it becomes necessary to use an anxiolytic, sedative, or analgesic, the lowest dose of the safest medication for the briefest period of time should be used. This plan will prevent a pill becoming a substitute for a relationship. Demands for medication will diminish as patients begin to feel secure with the physician/patient relationship. Physicians must realize that they cannot cure these patients. Listening and empathetic understanding is the best management. Physicians gradually help patients return to more normal life with such statements as, "You must be pleased to be able to go to the ballgame despite your pain and discomfort." Soon patients begin to talk about more than their physical symptoms.

Patients with somatization disorder have a lifelong illness. Nonetheless, a good physician/patient relationship will prevent unnecessary examinations, rehospitalizations, and inappropriate medications. Gradually the patient will be able to function better at home and at work.

Hypochondriasis

Hypochondriasis is a chronic condition characterized by a preoccupation with bodily function and an unshakable belief that physical illness is present. Although similar to patients with somatization disorder, patients with hypochondriasis lack the multiplicity of symptoms or the early onset of illness characterized by a somatization disorder. These patients dwell on their suffering and take over the interview.

A typical hypochondriacal patient is one who has chest pain. The patient will have a history of undergoing an exercise treadmill test, echocardiogram, cardiac catheterization, upper GI series, upper GI endoscopy, and will have been seen by a variety of cardiovascular surgeons and internists with no clear explanation of the symptom found.

When these patients are told of negative studies and reassured, their symptoms increase. Attempts at ameliorating their symptoms are met with a parodoxical response: their symptoms worsen, they develop side effects to the treatment, and they complain more. In a very uncanny way, these patients' complaints and symptoms decrease by acknowledging their sickness.

Treatment. The guidelines for treating patients with hypochondriasis are similar to treatment of somatization disorder (Table 14-5). The first goal is for the physician to redefine his own therapeutic goal. The physician should extinguish the goal of trying to abolish the patient's symptoms. One should listen objectively as possible to evaluate the situation and then communicate to the patient how difficult it must be for the patient to cope in light of these "terrible" medical problems. A general

Table 14-5. Hypochondriasis: Treatment

Redefine your therapeutic goals.
Listen, then communicate how difficult it must be for the patient to cope in light of these multiple problems.
"Don't just do something, sit there."
Follow-up regularly.

guiding principle is "Don't just do something, sit there." Avoid the tendency to jump in with another invasive diagnostic test or another potentially toxic medication. Minimize medications, minimize invasive tests, and minimize surgical procedures.

The cardinal rule is to see these patients regularly. The last thing in the world the physician wants to do is to see these complaining, frustrating patients often. If one accepts the challenge of trying to help these patients, one must overcome one's own negative reaction to these patients and see them regularly. A hypochondriacal patient should not leave the clinic without an appointment in hand guaranteeing his return. With this return visit guaranteed, the patient has their ticket to return and will not develop a worsened symptom for reentry.

Conversion Disorder

Conversion disorder can be understood as the "conversion" of anxiety into a physical symptom. The symptom prevents awareness of internal psychological conflict (primary gain), and while allowing the patient to avoid a noxious activity or receive a benefit that would otherwise be unattainable (secondary gain). For example, after becoming angry with his employer, a man is prevented by a paralyzed hand from hitting his boss (primary gain) and allows him to receive a much easier work assignment (secondary gain).

Neurological deficit such as paralysis, blindness, or seizures are the most common conversion symptoms. Occasionally the autonomic nervous system is involved. Vomiting or pseudocyesis (false pregnancy) can be conversion symptoms.

Although estimates on the prevalence of conversion disorder vary, most investigators agree that as the sophistication of the population increases, occurrence of conversion symptoms decrease. Conversion disorders are more commonly found in the lower socioeconomic classes and the rural populations. Young adults have conversion symptoms more often than older individuals.

Etiology. Stress often precipitates conversion symptoms. Unrequited love, a failed marriage, fear of pregnancy, and sexual problems are frequent precipitants of conversion symptoms in women; diminished self-esteem or work problems may result in conversion reactions in men. Traumatic events such as war or natural disaster, or the recent loss of a loved one may contribute to development of a conversion symptoms. Occasionally the precipitating event may appear insignificant to others, but a conversion reaction develops because the situation has special meaning to the patient. A physically ill person with whom the patient has a close relationship often serves as a role model for the conversion symptom.

Psychodynamic theory proposes that conversion disorder results from a conflict between an unconscious desire and fear of the desire. This conflict produces anxiety that is then converted into a physical symptom. The symptom expresses the repressed wish while at the same time offering relief from the emotional conflict. In addition, the conversion symptom provides escape from an unpleasant event or allows an excuse for failure.

Differential Diagnosis. A diagnosis of conversion disorder should be entertained in patients with symptoms that are inconsistent with physical findings. Diagnosis of a conversion disorder requires that the symptom serve a psychologic purpose and temporarily relates to the onset or worsening of the symptoms.

Multiple sclerosis can be confused with conversion disorder. While multiple sclerosis has a fluctuating course with multiple neurologic deficits, a conversion disorder is usually limited to one anatomic area. Patients with somatization disorder in addition to having conversion symptoms, also have many other organic complaints and lifelong histories of sickness. Unlike the patient with a conversion disorder, the patient with hypochondriasis does not suffer loss of physical functioning. Symptoms of a malingering or factitious disorder are under conscious control of the patient, while conversion symptoms are involuntary and reflect unconscious conflicts.

Prognosis. A patient with a stable personality prior to the onset of conversion symptoms has a favorable prognosis, especially if the illness was precipitated by a traumatic event. The dependent patient, whose emotional needs can only be met by assuming the sick role, has a poor prognosis.

Treatment. Treatment of conversion disorder involves a multidimensional approach focused to explain the basis of the symptom and also to deal with the unconscious conflict. Conversion disorder can be effectively treated by helping the patient understand the unconscious conflict that produces the symptom. The symptom can be removed by hypnosis, suggestion, or persuasion in a nonthreatening environment. Psychodynamic psychotherapy can help prevent recurrences.

Psychogenic Pain Disorder

Psychogenic pain disorder can be viewed as being very closely related to conversion disorder. To be diagnosed as having psychogenic pain disorder, an individual must have prolonged and severe pain with the complaint of pain exceeding the physical findings. Psychological factors contributing to the pain may be evidenced by a temporal relationship between a psychological stress and the onset of pain, enabling the patient to avoid an unpleasant activity, and allowing the patient to get special attention. Treatment for psychogenic pain disorder is multidimensional with a heavy reliance on behavioral techniques for pain management (see Chapter 9) and physical therapy.

FACTITIOUS DISORDERS

Factitious disorders are distinguished by psychological or physical symptoms voluntarily produced by the individual.

Ganser Syndrome

Ganser syndrome is marked by voluntary production of symptoms that suggest an emotional disorder. There is no apparent gain from the symptom. Patients demonstrate childish, ridiculous behavior and speech when they are being observed, but behavior returns to normal when the examiner leaves the room. Answers to questions are patently absurd, but replies indicate that the individuals understand what is being asked. For example, when asked how many legs a dog has, the individual may answer "five." Ganser syndrome, an extremely rare condition, usually occurs in prisoners or other special groups.

Munchausen Syndrome

Munchausen syndrome, named after an eighteenth century German baron who rode around the countryside telling fantastic tales, is a much more common and serious disorder than Ganser syndrome. The cardinal feature of the disorder consists of self-induced physical symptoms to gain hospital admission. Common physical complaints include abdominal pain, hemoptysis, nausea, vomiting, rashes, and abscesses. Patients suffering from Munchausen syndrome demonstrate pathologic lying and enjoy talking dramatically about their illness. Their attention-seeking behavior disrupts the hospital ward. Demanding analgesics and sedatives, they actively pursue exploratory surgery. They rapidly leave the hospital against medical advice once their deception has been exposed, only to seek admission to another hospital within a few days. Some of these patients, known as hospital hobos, follow the seasons, visiting northern hospitals in the summer and southern hospitals in the winter.

There are various explanations for Munchausen's syndrome: these individuals may seek a relationship with a physician as a substitute for an impaired maternal relationship; others may be acting out a grudge against the medical profession; still other may use self-mutilation to assuage unconscious guilt; or illness behavior may be a learned response.

Although the prevalence of Munchausen syndrome is unknown, a visit to a hospital's record room generally reveals a thick file listing "professional patients." There is no successful treatment for this condition.

DEPRESSION AND GRIEF REACTIONS

Depression is an illness of high prevalence in the medical setting and occasionally patients with depression will have as their primary manifestations those of a somatic nature. As opposed to the somatoform disorders, the somatic symptoms of depression are generally biological. Insomnia, anorexia, weight loss, impotence, constipation, and no energy are symptoms commonly seen in depression and rarely in somatoform disorders. Also, depressions are recurrent and often resolve spontaneously, somatoform disorders are chronic.

The hallmark distinguishing these illnesses from the somatoform illness is the patient's mood. Depressed patients report a depressed, "blue," or sad mood, while patients with somatoform disorders more often report anxiety and tension, or worry. There are those depressed patients who minimize the mood component to their illness. These have been variously labeled; one that neatly describes them is "masked depression." Their mood changes are masked by their prominent somatic manifestations. In every patient in whom excessive concern is evident, depression should be considered.

Grief reactions are also associated with excessive somatic concern. The grief response can be viewed as divided into three phases: 1) Shock phase; 2) Preoccupation phase; and 3) Resolution phase. The shock phase begins immediately after the loss, and during this time the patient has a sense of numbed disbelief and cannot comprehend the reality of the loss. This phase gradually wanes and the patient enters the phase of preoccupation where they constantly relive experiences and memories of the deceased. During the shock phase, one may see throat tightness, crying, sighing, and abdominal emptiness. Later, during the phase of preoccupation, the patient may complain of insomnia, weakness, fatigue, and anorexia. Both phases 1 and 2 have prominent somatic manifestations.

In evaluating patients with excessive somatic concern, one should take a history of recent losses. It may be that their symptoms are manifestations of the grief reaction. It is not uncommon for patients to develop the phase 2 symptoms during holidays, the anniversary date of the death, or other significant events. These "anniversary reactions" are usually transient and resolve spontaneously.

Further Differential

Patients with anxiety disorder also have excessive somatic concern. Generally, these patients have symptoms related to autonomic overactivity or mediated through the sympathetic

Table 14-6. Anxiety Related Symptoms

dyspnea
palpitations
chest pain
choking, smothering
dizziness, vertigo, or unsteadiness
paresthesias
sweating
fainting
trembling, shaking
headache
abdominal cramps
diarrhea

nervous system. (Table 14-6). As opposed to the patient with the somatoform disorders, patients with anxiety-related symptoms generally are improved following an objective evaluation, an explanation, and reassurance. Patients with organic brain syndromes can also present with excessive somatic concern. The geriatric literature is filled with anecdotal reports of patients with early dementing processes presenting primarily with somatic complaints. Often the cognitive impairment can be overlooked or can be so well compensated by the patient that it is missed. In any patient with excessive somatic concern, especially in the elderly, one should consider an organic brain syndrome and perform a thorough mental status examination.

The differential of excessive concern also includes the psychoses. The predominant manifestation of schizophrenia especially early in the illness may be more of bizarre somatic complaints than a disturbance of thought content. In the younger patient with a family history of schizophrenia and excessive somatic concern, one should consider an incipient schizophrenic illness as a cause of their excessive somatic concern.

Table 14-7 outlines the eight cardinal questions in dealing with a patient with excessive somatic concern. These questions

Table 14-7. Excessive Somatic Concern

1. Is the patient depressed or grieving?
   If Yes—evaluate and treat depression/grief reaction.
2. Is the patient psychotic?
   If Yes—evaluate and treat psychosis.
3. Is the patient organic?
   If Yes—evaluate and treat the organic brain syndrome.
4. Are symptoms those of autonomic overactivity?
   If Yes—think anxiety disorder.
5. Is there a precipitant stress or primary gain?
   If Yes—think conversion/psychogenic pain.
6. Illness behavior begin before age 30?
   If Yes—think somatization disorder.
7. Is there secondary gain?
   If Yes—think factitious illnesses.
8. Is the course compatible with hypochondriasis?

should serve as a guideline to assist in the diagnosis of these patients so that appropriate therapy can ensue. These are not easy diagnoses to make and furthermore, these are not easy patients to treat. The essential feature for managing these patients appropriately rests on the establishment of a physician-patient relationship, without which these patients are refractory to intervention.

Bibliography

Altman, N: Hypochondriasis. In Strain JJ, Grossman S (Eds), *Psychological Care of the Medically Ill: A Primer in Liaison Psychiatry.* New York, Prentice-Hall, 1975.

Barsky, AJ: Patients who amplify bodily sensations. *Ann Intern Med* 1979; 91:63–70.

Diagnostic and Statistical Manual of Mental Disorders, 3rd ed. Washington, DC, American Psychiatric Association, 1980.

Kolb, LC: *Modern Clinical Psychiatry.* Philadelphia, W.B. Saunders, 1977.

Mulder, DW: Organic brain syndromes associated with unknown cause. In Freedman AM, Kaplan HI, Sadock BJ (Eds), *The Comprehensive Textbook of Psychiatry* (Vol. 1), 2nd ed. Baltimore, Williams & Wilkins, 1975.

Walker, JI: *Clinical Psychiatry in Primary Care.* Menlo Park, CA, Addison-Wesley, 1981.

Chapter 15

DEPRESSION IN THE MEDICAL PATIENT

Gail Lynn Shaw, M.D.
John I. Walker, M.D.

Depression is a disturbance of mood and affect. Major depression occurs at some point in the lifetime of 18 to 23 percent of females and 8 to 11 percent of males based on studies done in Europe and the United States.[1] A recently conducted study involving over 9,000 adults in three sites found that from 4.6 to 6.5 percent of the population had a clinically significant depressive illness during a 6-month period.[2] Depression can be either primary or secondary. Primary depression—a depression that is unrelated to physical illness—can be subdivided into major depression, cyclothymic disorder, dysthymia, or atypical depression, depending upon the presenting symptoms. Secondary depression—known as organic affective disorder using the *Diagnostic and Statistical Manual of Mental Disorders,* third edition *(DSM-III)* classification system—is caused by a specific physical condition. This chapter will distinguish primary from secondary depression, briefly discuss biological tests used to confirm the diagnosis of depression, and give guidelines for the treatment of depression.

Primary Depression

Major Depression

Major depression refers to a syndrome characterized by a persistent dysphoric mood with a predominantly sad, "blue," low, hopeless, or irritable mood, lasting at least 2 weeks, with at least 4 of the following 8 symptoms:

1. Change in appetite or weight
2. Sleep disturbance
3. Psychomotor retardation or agitation
4. Loss of interest in work, hobbies, or sex
5. Decreased energy
6. Feelings of guilt or worthlessness
7. Difficulty concentrating
8. Suicidal ideation.[1]

Additional criteria for diagnosis include excluding coexisting illnesses such as grief or bereavement, organic brain syndrome, schizophrenia or other psychiatric illnesses, and paranoid disorder. Depression may present with physical complaints, especially pain. Other symptoms seen include: gastrointestinal distress, headaches, weakness, and fatigue. These patients with physical complaints may have a normal mood and appearance which is referred to as a "masked depression."

> A thirty-eight-year-old woman travel agent went to her physician complaining of fatigue. Her review of systems revealed that she had lost interest in her job and had difficulty choosing the flights for her clients. In addition, she had decreased appetite with a 5-pound weight loss over the prior month without dieting, early morning awakening, and a diminished libido. Physical examination and laboratory studies were normal, and the patient was felt to have major depression. She responded well to tricyclic antidepressant therapy.

Major Depression with Melancholia

The additional features of anhedonia, the total inability to feel pleasure, and mood nonreactivity, the inability to respond to pleasurable stimuli, constitute the diagnosis of major depression with melancholia. Additional criteria include at least 3 of the following symptoms:[1]

1. A depressed mood, different from bereavement, which the patient has difficulty explaining.
2. Increased severity of depression in the morning.
3. Awakening at least 2 hours earlier than usual.
4. Extreme psychomotor retardation or agitation.
5. Significant weight loss or severe anorexia.
6. Overwhelming guilt.

> A fifty-five-year-old police officer was taken to his physician by his wife after 2 weeks of missing work. The patient stated that he had just not felt like going to work. He spoke very slowly, but admitted that for 6 months he had been feeling hopeless s and increasingly despondent. He had loss of appetite, with a 30-pound weight loss over the preceding 6 months. It took him several hours to fall asleep, and he would awaken around 2 a.m. and be unable to sleep. He no longer got any pleasure from his work and had refused all social events over the preceding 2 months. The patient felt that he had been a failure and had contemplated suicide. The diagnosis of major depression with melancholia was made.

Major Depression with Mood-Congruent Psychotic Features

Some patients with major depression may have psychotic symptoms. If their psychotic features focus on themes of guilt, personal inadequacy, nihilism, or they have delusions of poverty or severe physical illness, they are considered to have mood-congruent psychotic features. The case below demonstrates a mood-congruent psychotic depression.

A fifty-four-year-old wife of a successful attorney had long been active in community groups. Over the previous year, she gradually lost interest in her organizations. She eventually dropped all participation and stayed home from the meetings. She then began to have difficulty falling asleep, lying awake for several hours, and then after sleeping would reawaken early in the morning and be unable to return to sleep. She began staying in bed late, although she was not asleep. The household chores then became an overwhelming effort. She had no energy, had difficulty concentrating, and felt very worthless. She felt unable to face the morning. She lost interest in food and eventually quit preparing dinner for her family. She spent more and more time in bed, and her thoughts turned inward. She developed the delusion that she had been an inadequate wife and mother. Despite the fact that she and her husband were quite wealthy and had entertained grandly in the past, she became worried that they would be poverty-stricken and turned out of their home. Her husband confirmed that their financial status was secure, and the diagnosis of major depression with mood-congruent psychotic features was made.

Major Depression with Mood-Incongruent Psychotic Features

On rare occasion, major depression may be associated with mood-incongruent psychotic features such as delusions of passivity or persecution or auditory hallucinations with commentary features. The following case is illustrative:

A twenty-year-old college student was taken to the Student Health Service by her friends. About 3 months earlier, she had become withdrawn and no longer went to parties or ate out with her friends. She admitted to feeling low in spirits, crying easily, and feeling fatigued. She complained of difficulty sleeping and had lost 20 pounds in the 3-month period. She had been going to fewer and fewer classes and for the past week had attended none at all. When the patient was asked why she no longer attended class, she replied that whenever she attended class, she heard voices telling her that if she remained in the classroom, a nuclear explosion would occur, destroying the entire university. She had hallucinations at no other time, and her thought content was otherwise normal. The diagnosis of major depression with mood-incongruent psychotic features was made.

Dysthymic Disorder

Dysthymic disorder represents a depressive illness similar to, but less severe than a Major Depression. Symptoms must have been present, at least intermittently, for 2 or more years. The patients describe long periods of depressed mood, accompanied by difficulty falling asleep, low energy, or any of the nonpsychotic symptoms and signs present in major depression. They characteristically feel best in the morning and despondent in the afternoon and evening. This disorder frequently coexists with personality disorders, alcohol and drug abuse, or major depression in partial remission. One of the distinguishing features from Major Depression is the absence of the biological abnormalities characteristic of major depression. DSM-III criteria for Dysthymic Depression are as follows:[1]

1. The patient has had depressive symptoms for at least 2 years. There may be intervening periods of normal mood, but these do not last more than a few months at a time. Neither severity nor duration of symptoms meet criteria for Major Depression.
2. During the depressive episodes, the mood is depressed, and there is mild anhedonia.
3. Three of the following symptoms are present:

    insomnia or hypersomnia;
    low energy or chronic fatigue;
    feelings of inadequacy;
    diminished performance or concentration;
    social withdrawal;
    anhedonia;
    anger or irritability;
    lack of pleasure in response to praise;
    decreased activity;

pessimism;
tearfulness;
frequent thoughts of death or suicide.

A fifty-four-year-old schoolteacher mentioned during her annual medical checkup that she was tired of teaching. She stated that she had never really enjoyed teaching and the students were completely undisciplined. She also said she never had been happy in her marriage. Her children had moved away from home immediately after high school and never visited her. She had no outside interests and had a cold relationship with her husband. The diagnosis of Dysthymic Disorder was made.

Cyclothymic Disorder

Cyclothymic Disorder is characterized by a mild depression which alternates with periods of hypomania, continuously or intermittently, over at least a 2-year period. The symptoms are not of sufficient number, intensity, or duration to meet diagnostic criteria for either Major Depression or Bipolar Disorder.

The patient was a thirty-one-year-old male bank teller. He had changed jobs 4 times in the past 8 years. He complained of mood swings, with highs and lows. When he felt high, he had more than his usual amount of energy, required very little sleep, and had the urge to be more productive at work and felt more successful with women. These episodes would last from days to weeks. At other times, he felt despondent, with little energy, no interest in work, and socially unable to function. This pattern had been going on since his college years. The diagnosis of Cyclothymic Disorder was made.

Atypical Depression

The *DSM-III* describes Atypical Depression as inclusive of the remaining affective depressive illnesses. Those individuals with depressive symptoms who do not fit criteria for a specific affective syndrome are classified as Atypical Depression. Historically, Atypical Depression has been used to identify those patients with depressed mood, prominent anxiety or phobias, hysterical features and atypical vegetative symptoms of hypersomnia and increased appetite with weight gain. These patients have been shown to gain little benefit from electroconvulsive therapy. They may represent a heterogenous group combining both depressive and anxiety disorders.

Recently, some criteria for atypical depression have been established. These include those patients who meet criteria for major, minor, or intermittent depression, demonstrate mood reactivity even while depressed, and exhibit 2 or more of the following symptoms: overeating, hypersomnia, extreme lethargy or fatigue, and extreme sensitivity to rejection.[3]

Bipolar Disorder

Bipolar affective disorder is characterized by episodes of mania frequently alternating with depression. There are usually intervening periods of normal mood. The manic patient displays hyperactivity, pressured speech, and elevated mood. The DSM-III criteria for mania are as follows:[1]

1. Elevated, expansive, or irritable mood.
2. At least four of the following symptoms:
   a) Hyperactivity
   b) Flight of ideas or racing thoughts
   c) Pressured speech
   d) Grandiosity
   e) Decreased need for sleep
   f) Distractability
   g) Excessive involvement in potentially disruptive activities (buying sprees, reckless driving, sexual indiscretions, etc.)
3. Duration of symptoms at least 1 week.
4. No evidence of schizophrenia or other psychiatric illness.
5. Symptoms not due to organic brain disease.

Psychotic features may also be present.

A thirty-three-year-old married nurse's aide spent $500 on

a new beach wardrobe in October in Buffalo, New York. She began wearing the front buttons on her nurse's uniform open. Then, she went to work in a bikini complete with name tag and nurse's cap. The supervisor called her husband who brought her to medical attention. Review of the preceding months revealed a depressive episode which had resolved. The diagnosis of bipolar disorder, manic episode, was made.

SECONDARY DEPRESSION

Organic Affective Syndrome

Affective disorders are often associated with general medical illness or drug reactions. The mechanisms by which depression is produced in these conditions is largely unknown. The symptoms of depression or mania present in organic affective syndrome are indistinguishable from the primary affective disorders. The relationship between depression and medical illness has many facets as described below:[4]

1. The depression is a reactive response to the illness.
2. The primary affective disorder becomes apparent at the same time as the medical illness.
3. The patient has a predisposition to depression which is exacerbated by the stress of a medical illness.
4. The somatic manifestations of depression overlap with those of the medical illness. In this case, treatment of the medical condition may or may not alleviate all the somatic symptoms.
5. Medications treating the illness may have depression as a side effect.
6. Depression may be directly related to the illness.

In trying to assess which medical conditions are truly associated with depression, it becomes apparent that many studies in the literature are difficult to interpret due to methodological flaws in study design.

Endocrine disorders. Endocrine disorders are frequently cited as producing psychological disturbances with features of depressive disorders. Hypothyroidism may present with the nonspecific symptoms of lethargy, constipation, and cold intolerance. They may subsequently develop slowing of intellectual and motor activity, depressed appetite with a modest weight gain. With florid myxedema, they develop a dull, expressionless face, with sparse hair, periorbital puffiness, large tongue, and pale, cool, rough skin characteristic of hypothyroidism. In some situations, the psychiatric reactions may dominate the clinical picture. Replacement with Levothyroxine results in resolution of the symptoms. Hyperthyroidism may also be associated with psychiatric symptoms. Weight loss and nervousness are common presenting complaints. In the elderly "apathetic thyrotoxicosis" may be the presenting form of the disease. Prominent features include apathy and a detached depression. The following criteria are useful for the diagnosis of apathetic thyrotoxicosis:

1. Apathetic appearance.
2. A small goiter.
3. Depression, lethargy, or apathy.
4. Absence of exophthalmus.
5. Muscle wasting.
6. Marked weight loss.
7. Atrial fibrillation or heart failure.[5]

Hyperparathyroidism may be associated with symptoms, ranging from mild personality disturbances to severe psychiatric disorders. The patient may have a complaint which can be mistaken for psychoneuroses. The characteristic features include the absence of initiative or spontaneous activity, suicidal ideation, fatigue, memory impairment, irritability, anhedonia, depressed self-esteem, pessimism, and difficulty concentrating.[5,6] The depressive symptoms are directly related to the serum calcium concentration, especially above levels of 11 mg/dcl. In addition, the hypomagnesemia associated with the hypercalcemia may contribute to the depression. The syndrome can be reversed by hemodialysis.[5]

Dysfunction of the adrenal glands can be associated with significant depression. Addison's description of adrenocortical deficiency in 1855 described "general languor and debility, remarkable feebleness of the heart's action, irritability of the stomach, and a peculiar change of the color of the skin."[7] Consequently, the progressive fatigability, weakness, anorexia, nausea, vomiting, and weight loss may initially be confused with depression. Cushing's syndrome, described in 1932, is characterized by muscle weakness and fatigability in addition to the more typical findings. Profound emotional changes can occur, ranging from irritability or emotional lability to severe depression, confusion, or even frank psychosis, with suicidal thoughts. Exogenous steroid therapy can produce depressive symptoms, but elation is more common.

The association of diabetes mellitus to depression is primarily a reactive depression. However, it has been shown that depression can have a significant negative impact on diabetic control. Increased metabolic stability can be maintained when the depression is treated.[4] When diabetes is complicated by impotence, a full-blown depressive illness may develop with psychomotor agitation or retardation, vegetative symptoms, and suicidal ideation.

A recent hypothesis suggests that a melatonin deficiency may produce psychotic depression. Melatonin, which is synthesized in the pineal gland, may act on the locus ceruleus, either directly or through the dorsal raphe nucleus. It may act as a monoamine oxidase inhibitor. Melatonin is synthesized from serotonin, and if melatonin acts as a monoamine oxidase inhibitor, there would be enhanced degradation of serotonin, resulting in a continuing cycle of serotonin-melatonin deficiency. The ineffective neurotransmitter discharge occurs in the locus ceruleus and/or the dorsal raphe nucleus, resulting in depression.[8]

Estrogens and progesterone have been implicated in the depressive illnesses. However, there are no good studies in the literature to support this, with respect to premenstrual syndrome, menopause, or exogenous estrogens. The relationship between menopause and depression is hampered by methodological flaws, but appears largely to be a function of predisposition to depressive illness.

Cardiovascular disease. The cardiac patient may frequently manifest depression. Anxiety, depression, and delirium are frequently reported in patients following heart surgery.[9] Postcardiotomy delirium varies from 13 to 70 percent.[9] This incidence is much higher than that seen in patients undergoing thoracotomy for other procedures. The association extends when it was shown that preoperatively 27 percent of cardiac surgery patients had depressive symptoms, and this rose to 75 percent with postoperative mood disturbance.[9] This syndrome associated with cardiac surgery does not appear to be merely a reactive depression because of the marked feelings of worthlessness, psychomotor retardation, and suicidal ideation. The depressed mood is out of proportion to the degree of the losses.

Infectious diseases. Infectious diseases can present as a psychiatric condition. Infectious mononucleosis and infectious hepatitis may be characterized by asthenia, anorexia, depressed mood, pessimism, and decreased ambition. One study found 25 percent of patients with depressed mood, pessimism, loss of self-esteem, diminished libido, anorexia, sleep disturbance, and diminished ambition persisting up to 3 weeks following influenza.[6] Others have reported a period of asthenia persisting from 4 to 6 weeks after influenza.[6] It is unclear whether the psychological depression is a primary result of the viral infection or a secondary response. Neurosyphilis has long been known as "the great imitator." Tertiary syphilis may manifest from 5 to 20 years following the initial infection. Symptomatic neurosyphilis occurs in roughly 20 percent of asymptomatic, untreated patients.[10] Neurosyphilis may mimic any psychiatric disorder such as depression, dementia, mania, psychosis, or delirium. General paresis, the paretic neurosyphilis, is the most common form to present as a psychiatric syndrome. Typically, it is a dementing process with diminished judgment, speech impairment, memory loss, and behavioral abnormalities. One study found 20 percent of 91 patients with neurosyphilis had the presenting symptom of dementia. Depression was a major feature in 27 percent of patients with general paresis.[10] The general features of these patients with depression include slowed movement, quiet affect, suicidal ideation, the presence of melancholia, nihilistic delusions, and other vegetative symptoms. Pulmonary infection has also been reported to be associated with depressive symptoms.

Hematologic disorders. Depression may be a prominent symptom in pernicious anemia. The associated dementia or confusional state is commonly misdiagnosed as presenile or senile dementia rather than depression. Treatment with vitamin B12 is associated with resolution of the symptoms.

Metabolic disorders. Metabolic imbalance may manifest with depressive mood changes. Hyponatremia, hypokalemia, and hypomagnesemia have been associated with severe depression. Uremia may manifest as suicidal ideation, apathy, and depressed mood. The hereditary hepatic porphyrias may manifest with hysteria, depression, and psychoses. Depressive symptoms may also occur with heavy metal poisoning and nutritional deficiencies. Pellegra, a deficiency of niacin, can manifest as fatigue, insomnia, apathy, irritability, nervousness and depression. It may proceed to a frank delirium. In addition, folic acid deficiency has been associated with depression.

Neurologic disorders. There are several neurologic diseases which have depressive symptoms as a prominent feature. The most commonly encountered disorder is dementia, which must be distinguished from a pseudodementia. This differential diagnosis in the elderly is further complicated by the frequent coexistence of a dementia of organic etiology. The new onset of psychiatric symptoms with relatively rapid progression over a matter of months in an elderly patient with no previous history of psychiatric disorder, coupled with a fluctuating clinical course, should raise the physician's suspicions that an underlying organic problem may be contributing to the behavioral disorder. The distinguishing features between dementia and pseudodementia due to depression include a rather sudden onset of symptoms in pseudodementia compared to a very gradual, insidious onset with dementia. The depressed patient with pseudodementia is aware of his cognitive deficits and has many complaints. On the other hand, the patient with true dementia appears oblivious to memory deficits that are quite apparent to observers. The depressed patient frequently is sad or apathetic, whereas the demented patient often has a labile affect. Memory testing reveals the depressed patient to give a clear, detailed, temporally coherent account of the present illness and past lives. When asked specific questions, however, they frequently respond, "I don't know," and stress these answers as evidence of the dysfunction.

Demented patients employ a variety of strategies to conceal their dysfunction from others. The diurnal variation of symptoms is also reversed: the depressed patient feels worse in the morning, whereas the demented patient experiences nocturnal worsening of cognitive functions. The depressed patient also usually has sleep and appetite disturbances, guilt, low self-esteem, fatigue, and anhedonia, whereas the demented patient does not experience these. The depressed patient with pseudodementia may also often show profound inconsistencies in their deficits across different tasks. For example, a patient could recount recent and remote events in great detail and in correct temporal sequence, but when read a test questionnaire, she stated that she could not remember the questions long enough to respond. Depression responds well to antidepressant therapy or electroconvulsive therapy, whereas the dementia is irreversible[5,11] (See Table 15-1).

Table 15-1. Characteristics Distinguishing Pseudodementia from Dementia

Characteristic	Pseudodementia (Depression)	Dementia
Onset	Rapid	Gradual
Course	Rapid progression of symptoms	Slow progression of symptoms
Complaint	Cognitive dysfunction	Denies cognitive deficits
Mood	Sad, apathetic	Labile
Associated symptoms	Sleep and appetite disturbance	Usually none present
Competence	Cognitive losses inconsistent across tasks	Consistent deficit
Diurnal pattern	Worse in morning	Worse at night
Resolution	Responds to antidepressant therapy or electroconvulsive therapy	Irreversible

Other nervous system involvement associated with depression includes cerebrovascular accident. Depression is a specific neurologic complication in 70 percent of right hemispheric cerebrovascular accidents. The etiology of depression in stroke is a complex combination of the loss of control, fears of death, disfigurement, loss of physical function and sexual impairment, loss of dignity, dependency, separation from their usual environment, lack of rapid improvement, and actual physical damage to cortical tissue. Hippocrates noted a relationship between epilepsy and depression when he stated, "Melancholics ordinarily become epileptics, and epileptics melancholics; of these 2 states, what determines the preference is the direction the malady takes; if it bears upon the body, epilepsy, if upon the intelligence, melancholy."[12] The sudden depression of mood has been felt to be part of an epileptic aura or a prodrome. However, the mood change lasts longer than usual for an aura or a postictal automatism. Many studies do reveal a high incidence of depression kin patients with epilepsy. The type of depression is debated as reactive, versus endogenous. In the search for a common pathogenesis between epilepsy and depression, disorders of noradrenaline, dopamine, 5-hydroxytryptamine, and gamma-aminobutyric acid and malfunctioning of the hypothalamic-pituitary axis have all been implicated in both conditions. The treatment of depression in epilepsy is complicated by the effect of tricyclic antidepressants in lowering the seizure threshold.

Early manifestations of normal pressure hydrocephalus are often behavioral changes. Over the course of a few months, the patients gradually developed apathy, psychomotor retardation, forgetfulness, unsteadiness of gait, and falling without loss of consciousness. The patients may develop an agitated depression, anxiety, paranoid delusions, ideas of reference, visual hallucinations, sudden violent and self-destructive behavioral manners, as well as argumentativeness.[13] As many as 60 percent of patients undergoing shunt operation for normal pressure hydrocephalus show objective improvement. The importance of fully investigating the new onset of a depressive or dementing illness in a previously healthy patient is illustrated in a case of dementia secondary to cerebrotendinous xanthomatosis. This rare neurologic disorder characterized by deposition n of cholestanol in the central nervous system and Achilles tendons was seen in a fifty-year-old man who presented with a major depressive disorder associated with dementia. The patient improved with treatment with haloperidol and doxepin.

Major depression is also seen with multiple sclerosis and Wilson's disease. The occurrence of depression in Parkinson's disease has a prevalence rate of 37 percent during evaluation or within 1 year before evaluation. It is hypothesized that the depression is not only reactive but biochemically related to the disease. Dopamine and its major metabolite homovanillic acid, as well as serotonin and norepinephrine, are decreased in the brains of patients with Parkinson's disease. The decrease in these neurotransmitters may contribute to the depressive illness. There are at least 3 cases in the literature of patients with Parkinson's disease demonstrating improvement of their Parkinsonian symptoms in addition to their depression with electroconvulsive therapy.[14]

The final remaining relationship between central nervous system disease and depression involves the effects of brain tumors, both primary and metastatic. General changes in psychological functioning presenting as depression can be seen and may be due to increased intracranial pressure. A metastatic brain tumor may account for symptoms not typical for the primary neoplasm.[5]

Malignant neoplasms. It is popularly stated that malignancy can present as a new depression. Yaskin was the first to describe carcinoma of the pancreas presenting with psychiatric symptoms.[15] Fras et al. prospectively studied 46 consecutive patients with histologically proven carcinoma of the pancreas.[16] Seventy-six percent had psychiatric symptoms temporally related to the presence of a neoplasm. More than one-half of these patients reported only psychiatric symptoms as their first indication of the illness. In 26 percent of these patients, the symptoms were considered to represent a primary psychiatric disorder. The most frequent symptom was depression, and the mental symptoms preceded the first physical symptoms by a median interval of 6 months. Pomara and Gershon described a patient with depression, unresponsive to antidepressants and electroconvulsive therapy for 10 years. He subsequently was found to have a 38 gram mass in the head of the pancreas and underwent a Whipple procedure. The patient's depression subsequently improved.[17] Of note, a relationship between depression and other intra-abdominal neoplasms has not been found. In the continuing search to elucidate the possible relationship between depression and the subsequent development of a malignancy, a prospective study using the Minnesota Multiphasic Personality Inventory (MMPI) was administered to 2,020 middle-aged men. Seventeen years later, a significant association between death from cancer and previous depression scores was demonstrated.[18] Adjustment for age, tobacco use, alcohol use, occupation and family history of cancer did not change the statistical association. Smaller prospective studies have not shown a relationship between depression scores and subsequent cancer. Brown and Paraskevas hypothesized that the depressive illness in cancer patients may be due to immunological interference with the activity of serotonin.[19] They postulate that protein released from cancer cells could crossreact with central nervous system tissue, bind to receptors for serotonin and block them, thus resulting in a relative serotonin deficiency and a subsequent depressive symptomatology. Other reviews of the literature have reached the following conclusions:

"a. There is no evidence that cancer patients have an increased experience of emotional loss prior to their disease, while there is some support for increased emotional inhibition and hopelessness in patients who already have cancer;
b. There is no solid evidence that cancer patients have increased depression in a psychiatric sense when compared to other patients, relatives, or normal control groups;
c. Psychometric assessment of depression also does not indicate increased prevalence of pathologic depression in cancer patients, though there is some suggestion that mild elevation in depressive symptomatology may be prospectively related to cancer incidence."[20]

There is little argument that reactive depression is a common complication of cancer.

Drugs. Depression is listed as a side effect for over 200 drugs. Only a small proportion of the patients treated with a specific drug experienced depression, however. Those individuals who are genetically predisposed to depression or who have had a previous depressive illness are more likely to experience drug-induced depression. This becomes a particular problem in the elderly, probably because responsiveness to drugs is different due to changes in drug disposition. Preexisting cerebrovascular disease may also play a role in potentiation of drug-induced depression. Whitlock and Evans suggest that "Any drug depleting the levels of dopamine, noradrenalin and 5-hydroxytryptamine (5-HT) or drugs that augment the levels and availability of acetylcholine in the brain and drugs potentiating the activity of monoamine oxidase may in certain circumstances cause depression."[21] Ethanol is well known to cause a depression in some users following heavy bouts of drinking when the blood alcohol levels are falling. Heavy alcohol intake results in a fall in the levels of 5-hydroxytryptamine and noradrenalin in the brain, and the subsequent release of acetylcholine is inhibited while blood levels remain high. Barbiturate and nonbarbiturate sedatives and hypnotics have similar pharmacologic effects and withdrawal symptoms compared to alcohol.[21] In addition, ethanol, phenytoin, as well as phenobarbital may cause folate deficiency which in and of itself can cause depression. Benzodiazepines appear to reduce 5-hydroxytryptamine turnover while inhibiting the release of acetylcholine from the nerve terminals.[21] These biochemical changes can result in depression.

The evidence for depression secondary to analgesics and nonsteroidal anti-inflammatory drugs is weak. There is some evidence that withdrawal from morphine precipitates depression, probably due to change in acetylcholine balance. Phenylbutazone, indomethacin, and ibuprofen have been reported to cause depression. One study observed depression in 4 of 70 patients using indomethacin, one of whom became suicidal. However, another study compared indomethacin and aspirin and showed a comparable frequency of depression, approximately 0.9 percent.[21] Assessments of depression secondary to nonsteroidal anti-inflammatory agents is clouded by the underlying arthritis which may cause depression.

Withdrawal from stimulants and appetite suppressants has been associated with depression. Amphetamines block the uptake of noradrenaline and dopamine and inhibit their destruction by monoamine oxidase. Consequently, amphetamine withdrawal results in a relative decrease of available neurotransmitters, resulting in depression. Phenothiazines can produce a picture of endogenous depression. Multiple reports on fluphenazine enanthate or decanoate have established an associated depression.[21]

Several studies have suggested that depressive reactions in patients receiving antihypertensive drugs are significant. Since patients with hypertension may have a history of a depressive illness, it is difficult to establish causation. Reserpine was associated with depression in 20 percent of 724 patients. Reserpine deletes the brain 5-hydroxytryptamine, dopamine, and noradrenaline, and the incidence of depression appears to be dose related, with depression more unlikely under 0.25 mg a day.[21] There is a 6 percent incidence of depression in patients taking methyldopa. The inhibition of the decarboxylation of dopa and 5-hydroxytryptamine by methyldopa leads to a decrease in catecholamines in the central nervous system. Other antihypertensives which have been implicated include guanethidine and clonidine. Recent studies continue to support a small incidence of severe to moderate depression occurring in patients treated with beta-blocking drugs for hypertension.[21] Most depression associated with antihypertensives resolves when the drug is withdrawn.

Steroids have been related to both depression and euphoria. The depression is seen more often with endogenous steroids as with Cushing's syndrome, whereas the euphoria is seen more often with exogenous steroids. Oral contraceptives have been widely implicated in causing depression. However, more recent studies have put this in doubt. Oral contraceptives deflect tryptophan into the kynurenine pathway with a result in decrease of 5-hydroxytryptamine; this process is reversed by giving pyridoxine.[21] Administration of pyridoxine improves depressive symptoms only in women documented to be Vitamin B6 deficient. Most women who develop depression on oral contraceptives have a previous history of depression.[21] A controlled study has failed to show any statistically significant increase in the incidence of depression in women taking oral contraceptives.

Antimicrobial agents have also been implicated in depressive symptoms. Older sulphonamides are strongly associated with depression, although this may be secondary to folate deficiency.[21] Cycloserine and isoniazid are also mentioned as causing depression, but they too may be related to folate deficiency. Metronidazole and griseofulvin have also been implicated to cause depression. Lysergic acid (LSD) diminishes 5-hydroxytryptamine turnover in the brain and inhibits brain acetylcholine esterase. It has been reported to cause depression in 15 of 70 patients.[21]

Parkinson's disease is well known to cause depression, but some patients appear to develop a more severe depression when treated with L-dopa or amantadine.[21] Disulfiram was reported to cause severe depression in 19 of 52 patients, with adverse reactions. This may be secondary to the action of disulfiram on dopamine-beta-hydroxylase, resulting in reduced levels of brain noradrenaline.[21]

The mechanism by which immunosuppressants and antineoplastic drugs may cause depression has not been well studied. Folate depletion may participate in this presentation.

Confusion and depression and other psychological disturbances may be seen with digitalis and digoxin or procainamide.[21] In summary, in the evaluation of depression, it is important to assess medications as possible etiologic agents. However, predisposition to depression, cerebral impairment, and serious disease make their own contribution to any depressive reactions noted.

DIFFERENTIAL DIAGNOSIS

Bereavement

Primary and secondary depressions must be distinguished from bereavement. The acutely bereaved may develop a sad mood with associated vegetative symptoms of sleep and appetite disturbance, fatigue, diminished libido, and anhedonia. This is a normal human response to a loss. Grief reactions can be overwhelming and lead to suicidal thoughts and actions. If the mourning extends longer than several months, then the illness becomes a major depression, and psychiatric treatment is indicated. The following case example is illustrative:

> A thirty-three-year-old man was brought to the ER by coworkers after threatening to take his life. The patient's wife had been killed in an automobile accident 3 months earlier, leaving him with 2 small children. Since her death, the patient had lost interest in life, in his work, and became anorectic with a 10-pound weight loss. He was unable to sleep at night and felt that life was no longer worth living. Work had become difficult due to impaired concentration. Crisis oriented psychotherapy was begun, and the patient's status improved over the following 2 months.

Anxiety

Anxiety disorders can be confused with depression because of the motor tension, emotional lability, and sleep disturbance that are commonly seen. Other features more typical of anxiety include an autonomic hyperactivity, apprehension, and hyperattentiveness. Features more consistent with depression would be the dysphoric mood, loss of interest in usual activities, weight loss, diminished libido, feelings of worthlessness and indecisiveness. The psychomotor agitation that can be seen with depression is not unlike the motor tension seen with anxiety disorders. The following case illustrates a patient who complains of anxiety, but who has biologic signs of depression and who should be diagnosed as depressed.

> A thirty-five-year-old administrative assistant complained to her physician of anxiety, tension, worry, and nervousness. Her symptoms were exacerbated by increased work load and the pressure of competing for a promotion. Further questioning revealed the patient had decreased appetite with a 10-pound weight loss over 3 months, decreased libido, frequent nocturnal awakening, and fatigue. This patient responded well to a tricyclic antidepressant.

The next case represents an isolated anxiety disorder:

A twenty-eight-year-old schoolteacher complained of increasing anxiety at school. She was unable to remain seated while her students were working on tests and found it necessary to walk around the room. When challenged with difficult discipline problems, she frequently became on the verge of tears. She had feelings of impending doom, edginess, restlessness, and fatigue. She was easily startled, and had difficulty falling asleep, but once asleep, slept well. This patient was felt to be suffering from an anxiety disorder and was managed with relaxation techniques and psychotherapy.

Laboratory Aids in the Diagnosis of Depression

The clinical history and examination of the patient are the most important step in diagnosing endogenous major depressive disorder. The dexamethasone suppression test is highly specific in most psychiatric disorders. The sensitivity ranges from 40 to 67 percent with a specificity of 96 percent. The positive predictive value of the dexamethasone suppression test is 80 to 94 percent. Disease prevalence has a well-known influence on the predictive value of a laboratory test, and thus the dexamethasone suppression test should be reserved for populations selected by clinical evaluation as probably having the disease. Since the dexamethasone suppression test is fairly specific for major depression, it should be negative in other psychiatric disorders and organic affective syndrome. It has been suggested that persistence of a positive dexamethasone suppression test indicates a greater chance of relapse.

The thyroxine releasing hormone stimulation test separates patients with major depression from minor depression. Its sensitivity is 25 percent, but its specificity is 75 to 93 percent. Consequently, its predictive value is low.

The biochemical theories of depression led to the development of the MHPG (3-Methoxy-Hydroxy-Phenylglycol) test. MHPG is the major metabolite of brain norepinephrine, and 20 to 60 percent of urinary MHPG comes from this source. A low urinary MHPG is associated with responsiveness to the norepinephrine antidepressants: imipramine or desipramine. A normal to increased urinary MHPG is associated with a responsiveness to serotonergic antidepressants such as amitriptyline.

The dextroamphetamine challenge test involves a patient interview, followed by 30 mg of oral dextroamphetamine with a follow-up interview. Improvement in the patient's depressed mood or psychomotor retardation is felt to be a positive dextroamphetamine challenge test which is correlated with a therapeutic response to noradrenergic antidepressants such as imipramine or desipramine.[22,23]

TREATMENT OF DEPRESSION

Pharmacologic treatment of major depression involves the use of tricyclic antidepressants, monoamine oxidase inhibitors, and lithium carbonate. The tricyclic antidepressants are usually the treatment of choice for major depression and depressive episodes of bipolar disorder. Their three major pharmacologic actions include:

1. Sedation.
2. Peripheral and central anticholinergic action.
3. Blockade of the "amine pump."[24]

The most sedating tricyclic antidepressants include the tertiary amines: doxepin, amitriptyline, and imipramine. The secondary amine tricyclics are somewhat less sedating: desipramine, nortriptyline, and protriptyline. It is important to prescribe therapeutic doses of tricyclic antidepressants in order to attain clinical benefit. In addition, it must be remembered that the tricyclic antidepressants take 2 to 3 weeks to exert their antidepressant action.

Monoamine oxidase inhibitors block the metabolism of brain norepinephrine, dopamine, and serotonin, resulting in an increase at the presynaptic level. Phenelzine, isocarboxazid and tranylcypromine seem to possess antidepressant, antianxiety, and antiphobic properties. This accounts for the usefulness of monoamine oxidase inhibitors in atypical depression. The side effects of hypotension from the medication or hypertensive crisis when tyramine-containing foods or drinks are taken with monoamine oxidase inhibitors have resulted in reluctance to use monoamine oxidase inhibitors. Consequently, they are used in patients refractory to tricyclic antidepressants.

Other medications used in the treatment of depression include antipsychotics for psychotic depression. The stimulant medications amphetamine, dextroamphetamine, and methylphenidate are ineffective in the treatment of depression and actually produce dependence and toxic paranoid psychosis. Similarly, benzodiazepines are ineffective in the treatment of depression.

Lithium carbonate is useful for acute manic episodes and the prophylactic treatment of manic and depressive episodes. Lithium is more useful in treating the depression of bipolar than unipolar illness. Close monitoring of its side effects and toxicity is necessary in lithium therapy.

Electroconvulsive therapy is more effective for treating depressive episodes than antidepressant drugs. Electroconvulsive therapy is indicated for those patients who do not respond to therapeutic levels of antidepressant medications and for those patients sufficiently dangerous to themselves to require treatment more rapidly than medication.[1]

Psychotherapy is useful in the acute management of the depressive episode in conjunction with medication. Several different modalities are available: psychoanalysis, psychodynamically oriented individual psychotherapy, cognitive therapy, group therapy, family therapy, and behavior therapy. Once acute symptoms have subsided, psychotherapy may focus on the underlying issues in the patient's life.

Summary

Depression is an illness commonly encountered by all physicians. It is critical to distinguish primary depression from secondary depression, due to underlying medical illnesses. Once this distinction has been made, appropriate therapy can be initiated.

References

1. *Diagnostic and Statistical Manual of Mental Disorders*, 3rd ed. Washington, DC, American Psychiatric Association, 1980.
2. Myers JK, Weissman MM, Tischler GL et al: Six month prevalence of psychiatric disorders in three communities. *Arch Gen Psychiatry* 1984; 41:959–967.
3. Leibowitz MR, Quitkin FM, Stewart JW et al: Phenelzine vs. imipramine in atypical depression. *Arch Gen Psychiatry* 1984; 41:669–677.
4. Lustman PJ, Amado H, Wetzel RD: Depression in diabetes: A critical appraisal. *Comp Psychiatry* 1983; 24:65–74.
5. Salzman G, Shader RI: Depression in the elderly. I. Relationship between depression, psychologic defense mechanisms and physical illness. *J Am Geriatrics Soc* 1978; 26:253–260.
6. Sachar EJ: Evaluating depression in the medical patient. In: Strain JJ, Grossman S (Eds). *The Psychological Care of the Medically Ill: A Primer in Liason Psychiatry*. New York, Appleton-Century-Crofts, 1975.
7. Addison T: *On the Constitutional and Local Effects of Disease of the Suprarenal Capsules*. London, Highley, 1855.
8. Maurizi CP: Disorder of the pineal gland associated with depression, peptic ulcers, and sexual dysfunction. *South Med J* 1984; 77:1516–1518.
9. Levenson JL, Friedel RO: Major depression in patients with cardiac disease: Diagnosis and somatic treatment. *Psychosomatics* 1985; 26:91–102.
10. Rundell JR, Wise MG: Neurosyphilis: A psychiatric perspective. *Psychosomatics* 1985; 26:287–295.
11. Wells CE: Pseudodementia. *Am J Psychiatry* 1979; 136:895–900.
12. Lewis AJ: Melancholia: A historical review. *J Ment Sci* 1934; 80:1–42.
13. Rice E, Gendelman S: Psychiatric aspects of normal pressure hydrocephalus. *J Am Med Assoc* 1973; 223:409–1412.
14. Asnis G: Parkinson's disease, depression and ECT: A review and case study. *Am J Psychiatry* 1977; 134:191–195.

15. Yaskin JC: Nervous symptoms as earliest manifestations of carcinoma of the pancreas. *J Am Med Assoc* 1931; 96:1664–1668.
16. Fras I, Litin EM, Pearson JS: Comparison of psychiatric symptoms in carcinoma of the pancreas with those in some other abdominal neoplasms. *Am J Psychiatry* 1967; 123:1553–1562.
17. Pomara N, Gershon S: Treatment-resistant depression in an elderly patient with pancreatic carcinoma case report. *J Clin Psychiatry* 1984; 45:439–440.
18. Shekell RB, Raynor WJ, Ostfeld AM et al: Psychological depression and 17-year risk of death from cancer. *Psychosomatic Med* 1981; 43:117–125.
19. Brown JH, Paraskevas F: Cancer and depression: Cancer presenting with depressive illness: An autoimmune disease? *Br J Psychiat* 1982; 141:227–232.
20. Bieliauskas LA, Garron DC: Psychological depression and cancer. *Gen Hosp Psychia* 1982; 4:187–195.
21. Whitlock FA, Evans LEJ: Drugs and depression. *Drugs* 1978; 15:53–71.
22. Fawcett J, Siomopoulos V: Dextroamphetamine response as a possible predictor of improvement with tricyclic therapy in depression. *Arch Gen Psychiatry* 1971; 25:247–255.
23. Van Kammen DP, Murphy DL: Prediction of imipramine antidepressant response by a one-day, D-amphetamine trial. *Am J Psychiatry* 1978; 135:1179–1184.
24. Hollister LE: Tricyclic antidepressants. *N Engl J Med* 1978; 299:1106–1109, 1168–1172.

Chapter 16

THE MEDICAL EVALUATION OF PSYCHIATRIC DISEASE

Ann Weisler Edmundson

One of the most difficult areas in medicine is the medical evaluation of psychiatric disorders. It is the fear of both psychiatrists and internists that a case diagnosed as depression, for example, and so treated, may in fact be due to a physical condition such as hypothyroidism.

The frequency of physical conditions totally responsible for or exacerbating psychiatric illness has been evaluated by several studies. In a survey of 2095 in-patients in a psychiatric hospital 18 percent of the patients had a medical illness totally responsible for their psychiatric diagnosis.[1] Similarly, in an out-patient series of 658 patients this figure was 9.1 percent.

This chapter will discuss three common psychiatric disorders—dementia, anxiety and depression—and the medical conditions that may cause them or may be confused with them. A guide to a medical evaluation of each disorder will also be presented.

Dementia

Dementia is a sustained decline in intellectual function secondary to a chronic disease process. The patient becomes disoriented in person, time, and place; he has difficulty recalling past events—recent more than remote—learning new tasks, and following simple verbal and written commands. Speech may become vague and incomprehensible. Confabulation may be a prominent feature, as in Wernicke-Korsakoff psychosis. Premorbid personality traits tend to become exaggerated. For example, patients with obsessive personalities may begin to keep lists. The patient's awareness of his declining intellectual abilities may result in depression and anger.

The cause of dementia in 417 cases evaluated at a university hospital is presented in Table 16-1.[3] The most common cause

Table 16-1. Causes of Dementia

	Number of cases	Percentages
Physical		
Intracranial Masses	20	4.8
Posttraumatic, Subdural	7	1.7
Normal Pressure Hydocephalus	25	6.0
Chemical		
Alcohol	42	10.0
Drugs	10	2.4
barbituates, opiates, lithium, bromides, heavy metals, volatile substances, etc.		
Hormone Defiency		
Hypothyroidism,*		
hypoparathyroidism		
Vitamin Deficiency		
B1 (Wernicke-Korsakoff), B12,*		
Folate		
Organ Failure		
Hepatic, Renal, Pulmonary		
Vascular		
Multi-infarct	39	9.4
Subarachnoid hemorrhage,*	28	6.7
Hypoxia*		
Hypertensive encephalopathy		

Table 16-1. Causes of Dementia *(continued)*

	Number of cases	Percentages
Degenerative		
Alzheimer's	199	47.7
Picks		
Huntington's chorea	12	2.9
Multiple sclerosis, Parkinson's,		
Creutzfelt-Jakob, Wilson's		
Infective		
Cerebrovascular syphilis, Cerebral		
tuberculosis, Abcess, Encephalitis*		
Inflammatory		
Temporal arteritis		
Systemic lupus erythematosis		
Polyarteritis nodusum		
Pseudodementia	23	5.5
Schizophrenia, Affective Disorders		
No Diagnosis	11	2.6

*Included in the causes listed as Subarachnoid Hemorrhage.

of dementia is Alzheimer's disease, which is characterized by diffuse cerebral atrophy of unknown etiology. An examination of the remaining causes in Table 16-1 reveals that many of the diseases have dementia as just one of their many symptoms and in these diseases rarely presents alone or as the first symptom. However, a demented patient may not be able to give an accurate history of his symptoms and it is important that the history also be obtained from family members. Particular attention should be given to a history of drug or alcohol use; family history of Alzheimer's, Wilson's, or Huntington's chorea; past history of syphilis, tuberculosis, anemia, hypertension, or thyroid disease; and a history of a fall or urinary incontinence.

    In the physical examination particular attention should be given to any evidence of other neurological problems such as ataxia in normal pressure hydrocephalus and focal neurological signs suggesting a space-occupying lesion such as a tumor, abscess or subdural. Often dysphasia or depression is confused with dementia and therefore special emphasis must be given to testing speech and determining affect. Some of the more common or confusing medical conditions are discussed below.

Normal Pressure Hydrocephalus

Normal pressure hydrocephalus is usually idiopathic but can result from trauma, chronic meningitis or subarachnoid hemorrhage. The course of the disease is variable but may be rapidly progressive. The diagnosis is suggested by a triad of symptoms: dementia, unsteady wide-based, short-stepped gait and urinary incontinence. The diagnosis is generally confirmed by computerized tomography of the head, which shows enlargement of the ventricles without cerebral atrophy.

Chronic Subdural

There is frequently no history of trauma or, if so, it is often trivial. Several weeks may elapse before the patient develops headache, slowed thinking or confusion. The patient often has a disturbance of consciousness which may be more prominent than localizing signs. The diagnosis is confirmed by computerized tomography of the head.

Hypothyroidism

The patient often exhibits a gradual decline in both physical and mental functions. Symptoms, in addition to mental sluggishness, include fatigue, hypersomnia, cold intolerance, constipation, weight gain, hoarseness and depression. Physical examination reveals an expressionless face, dry skin, myxedema and delayed and exaggerated tendon reflexes. The diagnosis is easily confirmed by a thyroid panel and thyroid stimulating hormone level.

Pernicious Anemia

Symptoms and signs of pernicious anemia affect the gastrointestinal tract, the nervous system and the blood. The patient may complain of a sore tongue which on exam will be smooth and red. Weight loss and diarrhea may also occur. Peripheral neuropathy, subacute combined degeneration of the cord, and disturbance in mentation may be present; the former two commonly preceding dementia. Examination of the peripheral blood smear reveals a macrocytic anemia with hypersegmented neutrophils. B12 level, Schilling's test and bone marrow examination confirm the diagnosis. Occasionally a patient may have neurological symptoms or even dementia alone with a normal hematocrit; therefore a B12 level should be included in addition to a complete blood count in the evaluation of dementia.

Multi-Infarct Dementia

This diagnosis is suggested by a history of hypertension, diabetes mellitus, or vascular disease. The patient often has a stuttering decline in intellectual function accompanied by other neurological symptoms. Computerized tomography of the head reveals areas of infarct.

Pseudodementia

Pseudodementia is a decline in intellectual function secondary to a psychiatric disorder. It is often hard to distinguish between pseudodementia and dementia and all too commonly this distinction is made only when a patient thought to be suffering from dementia recovers.
In a study done on 106 consecutively admitted patients with a diagnosis oof pre-senile dementia, 9.6 percent of the patients suffered from pseudodementia.[4] In the study above of 417 cases with dementia, this figure was 5.5 percent.[3]
The diagnosis is primarily made by clinical features. Table 16-2 lists some of the important features that differentiate between dementia and pseudodementia. Psychological testing with organicity usually distinguishes the two and identifies a psychiatric illness. In general, the medical work-up described in Table 16-3 is negative; however, minimal cerebral atrophy may be present in a patient with pseudodementia. It is only when the

Table 16-2. Features Distinguishing Pseudodementia from Dementia

	Pseudodementia	Dementia
Onset	may be sudden	gradual
Prior psychiatric history	common	occasionally
Memory loss	remote more than recent, often specific	recent more than remote
Performance of tasks	variable	consistently poor
Answers to questions	"don't know"	near-miss
Social skills	lost	preserved
Perception of inabilities	emphasizes loss	minimizes
Affect	depressed and distressed	shallow, labile

dementia is out of proportion to the small degree of cerebral atrophy and the clinical picture fits pseudodementia that Alzheimer's disease may be excluded. It should be noted that the degree of dementia does not always correlate with the degree of cerebral atrophy. In a study of the brains of demented patients it was found that minimal cerebral atrophy could be present in significantly demented patients.[5]

Table 16-3 lists the diagnostic tests helpful in identifying the cause of dementia.

ANXIETY

Anxiety is a subjective feeling of uneasiness and apprehension out of proportion to the perceived threat. It is one of the most common complaints made by patients. It can take many forms: constant, intermittent over a period of days, or panic attacks, lasting several minutes, when a patient is suddenly filled with a sensation of impending doom or loss of control. A wide range of somatic complaints may accompany anxiety, including

Table 16-3. Diagnostic Tests in the Evaluation of Dementia

	To Diagnose
Hematology	
Complete blood count	Macrocytic anemia, infection
Folate, B12	Deficiency
Serology	
VDRL	Cerebrovascular syphilis
Chemistry	
Electrolytes, Blood urea nitrogen, Creatinine	Pulmonary, renal, endocrine disorders
Bilirubin, Transaminases	Liver disease
Thyroid panel, TSH	Hypothyroidism
Arterial blood gas	Pulmonary or metabolic derangement
Drug levels	When appropriate
Radiology	
Chest roentgenogram	Infection, tumor, or other lung disease
Head computed tomography	Tumor, subdural, normal pressure hyrocephalus, multi-infarct dementia
Procedures	
Lumbar puncture	Meningitis, cerebrovascular syphilis, tumor
Psychological testing and organicity	Confirm diagnosis, pseudodementia

headache, shortness of breath, palpitations, chest pain, tremor, fatigue, gastrointestinal disturbances and perspiration.

Anxiety, as part of a psychiatric diagnosis, commonly affects females more often than males. It usually begins in adolescence or early adulthood and seldom occurs for the first time after age thirty.

In distinguishing the various causes of anxiety, particular attention should be given to previous psychiatric history; alcohol or drug use; symptoms and signs of hormonal abnormalities; cardiac or central nervous system disease; and family history of epilepsy, porphyria, or endocrine or psychiatric disease. The causes of anxiety are listed in Table 16-4.

Some of the medical conditions that may cause anxiety include:

Hyperthyroidism

Hyperthyroidism not infrequently presents as anxiety in a young patient. Many of the manifestations of psychiatric anxiety are indistinguishable from those of anxiety due to hyperthyroidism, viz. fatigue, irritability, restlessness, diarrhea, weight loss and palpitations. The distinguishing features of hyperthyroidism are the absence of previous psychiatric disease and anorexia; and the presence of thyroid prominence, eye signs, skin changes such as onycholysis, and cardiac abnormalities like atrial fibrillation. The diagnosis is confirmed by thyroid function tests.

Table 16-4. Causes of Anxiety

Chemical
  Alcohol withdrawal
  Drugs
    Amphetamines, sympathomimetic, atropine, caffeine, cocaine, glue, LSD, lead, barbituate withdrawal
  Hormonal
    Hyperthyroidism, hyperadrenocortism, pheochromocytoma, carcinoid, hyper/hypoparathyroidism, hypoglycemia
  Biosynthesis
    Porphyria
Vascular
  Pulmonary embolus, internal hemorrhage
Cardiac
  Mitral valve prolapse, arrythmias, impending myocardial infarct
Neurological
  Post-concussive, complex partial seizures, encephalitis
Psychiatric
  Depression, neurosis, schizophrenia

Pheochromocytoma

Although a rare disorder, pheochromocytoma enters into the differential diagnosis of panic attacks. The clinical manifestations are secondary to catecholamine excess and consist of headache, blurred vision, perspiration, palpitations, tremor and paroxysmal or persistent hypertension. Orthostatic hypotension often ensues secondary to atrophy of the usual sympathetic postural reflexes. Initial evaluation includes 24 hour urine for vanillylmandelic acid, catecholamines and metanephrines.

Mitral Valve Prolapse

A patient with mitral valve prolapse may present a wide array of symptoms including atypical chest pain, syncope, palpitations and anxiety. Most patients, however, are asymptomatic. It occurs more frequently in young females, and echocardiograms of random young females show the prevalence to be as high as 10 percent. It is therefore not clear whether symptoms as vague as anxiety are referrable to mitral valve prolapse. It is suggested that some of the symptoms experienced in mitral valve prolapse are secondary to autonomic dysfunction. The diagnosis is suggested by a mid to late systolic click and or a systolic murmur in the mitral area and is confirmed by echocardiogram.

Complex Partial Seizures

Complex partial seizures are characterized by psychic auras consisting of illusions, hallucinations, alterations of reality or change in affect. The aura may occur alone or be followed by a period of unresponsiveness or automatism for which the patient is amnesic. The seizure may then become generalized. Such a seizure might cause the patient to experience an unusual smell; burning rubber, for example, extreme anxiety and lip smacking. It is the repetition of the aura and the lack of relation to external reality that helps distinguish complex partial seizures from panic attacks.

The diagnosis is confirmed by the spike or slow wave discharges in the temporal region of an EEG. A normal EEG does not exclude the diagnosis. Nasopharyngeal or sphenoidal electrodes enhance the sensitivity of the EEG by recording deeper in the temporal lobe but, even so, the focus may be so deep that the EEG may not detect the abnormality without more extensive studies. Some of the diagnostic tests that may be useful in an evaluation of anxiety are listed in Table 16-5. Clearly, the clinical situation determines which, if any, are indicated.

Table 16-5. Diagnostic Tests in the Evaluation of Anxiety

	To diagnose
Hematology	
Complete blood count	Infection, lead intoxication, anemia of chronic disease (e.g. hyperthyroidism)
Chemistry	
Electrolytes	Hyperadrenocortism
Calcium, phosphorus, albumin	Hyper/hypoparathyroidism
Glucose, Glucose tolerance test	Hypoglycemia
Thyroid function tests	Hyperthyroidism
Urinary VMA, catecholamines, metanephrines	Pheochromocytoma
Drug screen	As indicated
Radiology	
Chest roentgenogram	Cardiac abnormalities
Barium studies	Gastrointestinal complaints
Procedures	
EEG with nasopharyngeal leads	Complex partial seizures
EKG, Holter monitor	Arrythmias
Echocardiogram	Mitral valve prolapse

DEPRESSION

Depression is an exaggerated sadness and pessimism out of proportion to life's circumstances. The patient may also experience feelings of unworthiness, hopelessness, and guilt, may become lachrymose, suicidal, and may wish for death. Auditory hallucinations or delusions may also be present. Physiological symptoms such as early morning waking, fatigue, loss of weight

Table 16-6. Causes of Depression

Physical
  Subdural
Chemical
  Alcohol
  Drugs
    Anti-hypertensive medication: methyldopa, propanolol, reserpine
    Neuropsychiatric: barbituate, benzodiazepine, cessation of amphetamines or cocaine, disulfiram, levodopa
    Other: digitalis, steroids, thallium, carbon disulphide
  Hormones
    Cushing's, Addison's, Diabetes mellitus, hypoglycemia, Hyper/hypothyroidism
  Vitamin Deficiency
    B12
  Organ Failure
    Hepatic, renal, pulmonary
  Electrolyte Imbalance
    Hyponatremia, hypokalemia, hypercalcemia
  Degenerative
    Multiple sclerosis, Huntington's chorea, Alzheimer's, Pick's
  Infective
    Post-viral, infective mononucleosis, hepatitis, encephalitis, Cerebrovascular syphilis, cerebral tuberculosis
  Neoplastic
    Occult malignancy, cancer of the pancreas
  Psychiatric
    Schizophrenia, major affective disorder, bipolar affective disorder

and appetite, decreased libido, and constipation may also be prominent.

Depression may accompany any medical illness or surgical procedure, depending on the patient's personality and circumstances. However, in certain illnesses listed in Table 16-6, depression is the main or presenting feature.

In evaluating a patient with depression, inquiry must be made into the history of previous psychiatric disease including mania, family history of psychiatric disease, recent loss, such as death of a relative, medications, and alcohol use. In addition, questions must be asked to elicit the symptoms of the diseases listed in Table 16-6. Some of the causes of depression are listed below.

Drugs

A large number of drugs may cause depression. This is a very difficult diagnosis to make and it is only after the drug has been stopped and the patient then re-challenged that the diagnosis can definitely be made. Clearly, in many cases, drugs exacerbate an underlying psychiatric depression.

Drugs that commonly cause depression include several antihypertensive medications. Reserpine is well known for this complication. The biochemical mechanism is thought to be due to depletion of intraneuronal concentrations of serotonin, dopamine and norepinephrine. The other anti-hypertensive medications that produce depression are also felt to influence amine metabolism at the pre-or post-synaptic level.

Hypercalcemia

Depression may be a symptom of hypercalcemia. Other neurological symptoms include mild personality changes to severe obtundation, proximal muscle weakness and headache. In addition, hypercalcemia may affect the gastrointestinal tract, joints and bones, and kidneys. Once the diagnosis of hypercalcemia has been made, appropriate investigations, such as protein electrophoresis and parathyroid level, are in order, to determine the underlying cause.

268 THE COMPLICATED MEDICAL PATIENT

Occult Malignancy

Although an uncommon cause of depression, occult malignancy, in particular cancer of the pancreas, has been noted to present with depression. Generally depression of psychiatric cause begins in the fourth decade. The occurrence of depression in an elderly patient with no precipitating cause is suggestive of an organic cause. Table 16-7 lists some studies that may be informative in the evaluation of a depressed patient.

The three conditions discussed above; dementia, anxiety and

Table 16-7. Diagnostic Tests in the Evaluation of Depression

	To Diagnose
Hematology	
Complete blood count	Pernicious anemia, infection
B12	Pernicious anemia
Serology	
VDRL	Cerebrovascular syphilis
Monospot	Infectious mononucleosis
Chemistry	
Electrolytes, Blood urea nitrogren	Electrolyte imbalance, Cushing's, Addison's, renal, pulmonary
Glucose	Diabetes mellitus, hypoglycemia
Thyroid panel, TSH	Thyroid disease
Calcium, phosphorus, albumin	Hyperparathyroidism
Liver function tests	Liver failure, hepatitis
Drug levels	When indicated
Radiology	
Chest roentgenogram	Pulmonary disease, occult malignancy
Head computed tomography	Subdural
Procedure	
Lumbar puncture	Infection, if indicated
Dexamethasone suppression test	Major depression

depression are generally not secondary to a treatable organic cause. It is important, however, that both psychiatrists and internists evaluate each patient with these problems from a medical point of view in the initial assessment.

REFERENCES

1. Koranyi EK: Morbidity and rate of undiagnosed physical illness in a psychiatric clinic population. *Arch Gen Psychiatry* 1979; 36:414–419.
2. Hall RC et al: Physical illness manifesting as psychiatric disease. *Arch Gen Psychiatry* 1978; 35:1315–1320.
3. Wells CE (Ed): *Dementia* (2nd ed). Philadelphia, Davis, 1977.
4. Marsden CD, Harrison MJG: Outcome of investigations of patients with presenile dementia. *Br Med J* 1972; 2:249–252.
5. Tomlinson BE, Blessed G, Roth M: Observations on the brains of demented old people. *J of Neurol Sci* 1970; 11:205–242.

Chapter 17

THE ILL PHYSICIAN

A Complicated Medical Patient

Conrad Fulkerson, M.D.

A variety of factors may complicate our patients' illnesses. Complications that come to mind include the almost infinite permutations of pathophysiology, illness superimposed upon illness, and exotic "high-tech" medicine that both treats and creates complicated patients.

Some patients are complicated not by the illnesses they present but rather by who they are personally, sick or well. Such is the case of the physician-patient. No other phenomenon in medical practice demonstrates quite as well the intricacies of the physician-patient relationship or reveals the impact and deep ramifications of that relationship. Few other issues in medicine are as difficult for us to consider as our own potential morbidity or the illness or disability of our colleagues.

An increasing body of literature concerns a condition termed the "impaired physician".[1,2] This designation is useful, since everyone, including physicians, have been so inclined to avoid recognizing the doctor who is unable to function professionally due to illness and/or substance use. This defined concept has permitted identification of a particular and painfully prevalent syndrome and encouraged at least a beginning dialogue among clinicians as well as licensing authorities, legal representatives, trainers and educators, and health care administrators.

With this recognition, troubling but crucially important information has become available. More than 100 physicians take their own lives each year (dramatically equated by some to the size of a medical school graduating class). While the debate continues[3] as to whether this represents a rate in excess of the general population, the fact itself is alarming enough.

Among physicians, narcotic addition is 30 to 100 times greater than in the general population.[4] Alcoholism and its sequelae are significantly increased[4,5] with some reports of physicians admitted to hospitals over twice as often as the general population for problem drinking.[6] When substance abuse and suicide rates are considered together, some have estimated that the equivalent of seven entire medical school classes is lost annually to medical practice.[7]

The general health of physicians on screening examinations does not seem to differ from similar nonphysician patients.[8] Fewer data are available regarding physicians' illnesses in general than in some specific areas (such as substance abuse). Seventy percent of doctors did not receive regular medical examinations in one study[8] and physicians have been found to delay seeking attention of symptoms suggesting cancer.[9]

There is, however, some recent evidence[10] that physician self-care may be better than suspected. A major study of physicians' health currently underway has shown low rates of tobacco use and high rates of dietary awareness and regular exercise among randomly selected participating doctors.

Though a direct continuum is difficult to trace, there is ample evidence to suggest that the alarming rate of disabling physician impairment and the general health care sought by and available to the physician are related. One impaired professionals program has compiled lists of characteristic behaviors of alcohol and drug-addicted physicians in six basic areas of living which are affected in sequence by substance abuse and found that the last area to show signs of impairment is the doctor's professional activity.[11]

It seems likely, then, that we are only dealing with the tip of the iceberg as the data accumulates regarding noticeably impaired physicians. Some urgency in viewing any ill physician as a complicated medical patient and seeking to better understand ourselves as patients seems well justified.

Just who is this "physician" who may, upon occasion, become a patient? This physician is a very important person who frequently suffers needlessly due to "VIP" treatment. This physician is most often a virtuous person whose virtue when carried to an extreme is a hazardous vulnerability. This physician is a hardworking person whose work can come to encompass personal identity and self-worth with vocation merging into blissful escape, merging into behavioral addiction.

Vaillant[12] painstakingly explored the childhoods of 47 physicians followed longitudinally for 30 years of adult life, and concluded that much of the doctor's vulnerability to substance abuse and marital discord could be accounted for by early life experience. Long-standing feelings of inferiority seemed more common among physicians, and Vaillant proposes that the opportunity to care for appreciative patients may attract persons from an emotionally barren childhood who may seek and receive emotional sustenance from medical practice. Furthermore, physicians were twice as likely to avoid asking for help and to avoid direct expression of emotions as matched controls. These doctors were inclined not to inconvenience others in order to meet their own needs.

Following childhood, aspiring physicians proceed over an increasingly harrowing series of hurdles including demanding academic performance, "personal development and well-roundedness" (known by applicants to be evaluated by admissions committees), and drills for medical college admissions tests that may include elaborate and expensive commercial tutoring. Clearly, only a highly motivated, if not driven and compulsive student, arrives even at the admissions process, not to mention the select subset that are taken as first-year students.

The role that medical school (with anticipation reaching back as early, these days, as junior high school) and postgraduate training have on the physician's future difficulty in accepting the patient role, when need be, is uncertain and controversial. It has been estimated that up to half of medical students need psychotherapy[13] but fewer receive it.

McCue[14] has written eloquently on the distress of the internship and raises the question whether the usual postgraduate training program is detrimental to physicians both by its demands at the time and the attitudes that it may instill for the future. Other critics of the internship[15] bluntly ask if it is a year of "preparation or hazing?"

Whatever the direct stresses of the internship and residency, the long hours and loss of sleep are forgotten and "surviving the internship takes on an almost ritualistic meaning."[14] Not forgotten, however, are the attitudes shaped during this time. An ongoing process whereby the future physician assumes a posture and identity of being unique, separate from others, independent, and of privileged status is accelerated. This identity is, indeed, deserved and earned. It is also quite necessary to be separate, apart, and embued with very special authority to function as a physician making difficult decisions made by no one else in society. The physician, and most intensively the physician in training, faces suffering, fear, sexuality, and death each day.[16] The distinction of subject (the doctor) and object (the patient), sickness and health, the functional and the dysfunctional, becomes sharper and sharper.[17] The doctor is not the patient; the patient is not the doctor. The contrasting and complementary roles of the authoritative physician and the patient in the patient role develop.

There are, however, some confounding twists in this process—a powerful, largely unconscious process, both individual and social. First, from the beginning of this long and arduous career path, a significant but usually covert assumption has constantly been present. This is the idea that one's very suitability to practice medicine is inherently dependent upon and measured by one's ability to survive and perform at the various levels of training. To be ill, to need time away, or to need more rest than is dictated by a call schedule suggests to the trainee (or may be suggested by program directors) that medicine just may not be for him. Just how realistic the program demands are is rarely questioned. The trial and challenge of training becomes both a selective process and a powerful influence on the young physician's attitudes, opinions, and identity.

A second factor operating during the training years and

continuing into professional life is the set of attitudes developed by others—colleagues, friends, family, and other health care professional and administrators—as to just what it means to be a physician. The comforting idea of the caring, curing, compassionate healer is as old as civilization itself. Originally, however, even the physician was expected to rely on God. It is only with the later split of biological from spiritual thinking that the *completely* reliable, omniscient, invulnerable physician has come to be expected by the physician himself, as well as by virtually all those around him.[17]

Finally, during this professionalization process, the virtues of the physician—altruism, selflessness, and dedication to others—are rewarded and developed further. While these aspirations, with their roots in early life, are frequently the foundation for even the earliest motivation to study and practice medicine and represent the best in human values, it is clear that their extension to the extreme can only further isolate the physician from potential sources of help for himself.

With the foregoing, the well-known fact that physicians are usually poorly prepared to be patients is even more understandable. When the physician becomes ill and begins to experience symptoms in his own body, the doctor is confused, alternately minimizing and catastrophizing this strange experience. Only occasional physicians have had much experience with illness prior to adulthood. Medical schools tend to prefer healthy, vigorous candidates and training programs select similarly. The physician's experience with illness and with being a patient is limited to playing a sharply contrasting though complementary role, that of the doctor.

The role of the patient, assumed as needed by persons for centuries has been "so utterly taken for granted that it had no name until 1951 when sociologist Talcott Parsons described it and called it the 'sick role' ".[18] Parsons's[19] description included the following: 1) the sick person may be relieved of usual responsibilities; 2) The sick person is not to blame for his illness; 3) the sick person is not expected to know what to do regarding his illness; and 4) the sick person is expected to accept the help of knowledgeable persons and to wish to get well.

The physician is unprepared to assume this patient role that so directly contrasts with his very identity and sources of self-worth. He experiences a crisis. When symptoms can no longer be denied, perhaps self-treatment is the answer. Numerous drug-dependent physicians relate such a history. Or perhaps the physician will approach another physician in the only way the knows: as a colleague.

The "hallway consultation" is familiar to all physicians, and much of the professional business of medicine seems to be conducted in corridors. Dlin[20] writes that through his career he has learned to take the casual remarks and inquiries of colleagues seriously. Tragically, this may be the only way in which an ill physician seeks help. The avoidance of asking for help is confounded by the response of many physicians to such casual inquiries from their colleagues. It may seem inappropriate to regard or speak to a colleague as a "patient." Seeing our associates suffer is frightening, making many of us aware of our own vulnerability. Dlin[20] writes, "When a colleagues stops me in the corridor to talk about a patient and then, with some genuine effort, manages to talk about himself or his family's problems, I make it my business to give him the opportunity to elaborate, either then or later." Even if this initial difficulty in seeking care is somehow traversed and the physician-patient enters the health care system, his care continues to be complicated. The medical care of the physician poses unique problems not only for the physician-patient but also for his physician(s) and other health care professionals that may be involved.

The physician-patient under medical care is faced with profound threats to his self-esteem and to his sense of authority, control, and responsibility by assuming the patient role. Physicians remain physicians, even when patients, in that they retain their medical knowledge and experience and are intimately familiar with the workings of the health care system. It is easy for the physician patient to remember laboratory reports that get lost, errors in X-ray, and all of those day to day failings of a complex medical center.

The physician is away from his practice (the schedule that he developed with the idea that he would never be ill) and, with his usual sense of responsibility and altruism, feeling guilt for the burden placed on his colleagues in his absence and the suffering of his own patients whom he is unable to attend. The physician has, in the past, equated illness or disability with total failure and has invested a tremendous amount of time, energy, and money in his career. He may feel that much or all is lost. With this experience of illness and forced into (or at least toward) an unfamiliar and uncomfortable role, the ill physician may become hostile, demanding, and controling[21] or he may withdraw, become depressed, and persist in not wishing to trouble or inconvenience others. He may be ashamed and embarrassed at being a patient.

For the attending physician with a doctor-patient, the task is similarly difficult and stressful. The physician may be uncertain as to what to explain to this medically sophisticated patient. He may deal only very superficially with issues, assuming (and perhaps hoping) that his patient will "understand" and he will not have to discuss embarrassing or unpleasant details. With today's degree of medical specialization, it is not uncommon for a very specialized treating physician to find that a similarly but differently specialized physician-patient is much more naive about his illness and its treatment than he had ever thought. The attending may in his discomfort with these complicated roles and relationships belabor his colleague-patient with detail or even attempt to maintain him as a colleague in his "case," relating to him more as a consultant than a patient.

The treating physician may feel "on the spot" and in conspicuous public view within the medical community where news of an ill associate spreads rapidly, albeit in hushed tones. To fail in the treatment of this "very important person" would, indeed, be a very public failure. Feelings such as these are an invitation to overtreatment and overevaluation lest something be missed.

The attending physician's own attitudes about personal illness cannot help but influence his treatment of his colleague and a tendency to overidentify with his patient is likely.[21] The physician may respond more to his own perceived needs and wishes (as if he were the patient) than clearly hear what his patient is telling him.

This physician and physician-patient relationship occurs in the context of other health care professionals, friends, family, and colleagues. Nursing, laboratory, and other clinic or ward staff are usually noticeably affected by the presence of a physician-patient. Many of the reactions that the attending physician experiences may occur with nursing staff. While the staff may respond to the physician-patient's own emotional reactions with escalating tension or hostility, the staff may react with hostility, resentment, or envy simply because their patient *is* a physician, and become determined to make the ill physician more of a patient than he needs to be.[22] These relationships may be even further confused if any of the staff has previously seen the ill physician as a patient themselves.

Despite the complexity of treating the ill physician and the abundance of points at which care may go astray, physicians are treatable patients and often learn a great deal themselves from the experience of being a patient.[18] Even with physicians ill to the point of professional impairment, the prognosis with treatment in informed and specialized settings is good. One drug and alcohol program found that upon follow-up, physician-patients had a significantly better prognosis than the general patient population.[23] The fundamental principles in approaching and treating the physician-patient are rooted in the powerful and complex role relationships involved. A great measure of the confusing emotions, garbled communication, and errors in diagnosis and treatment can be traced to insufficient appreciation of these crucial relationships. An appreciation of the patient or "sick" role and the corresponding role embodied in the physician's "Aesculapian authority" is delightfully gained from Siegler and Osmond[18] in their book *Patienthood: The Art of Being a Responsible Patient*. It is highly recommended and would be a fruitful assignment for the physician-patient as well as his doctor.

Our responsibility to ill colleagues begins when we are first approached by them even if the setting is informal or in a corridor. These requests should be tactfully handled and the inquirer should be gently steered to a more appropriate setting. Often the requesting physician will welcome such a response from a colleague and is hesitant to ask for more than "curbstone" time. Follow-up is crucial, especially if a referral has been made.[21]

Once the physician-patient is seen in an appropriate setting, the treating doctor should set about doctoring and allow the patient to become a patient with his due share of ignorance, fear, mistrust, uncertainty, questions, and reliance upon his physician for decisions. The crucial factor is the physician-patient relationship that develops and the clarity and comfort of communication that takes place. Early on, it is appropriate to acknowledge to the patient how difficult it can be to seek care, how worrisome illness may be ("even though we deal with it every day . . ."), and to express appreciation for the confidence placed in the colleague that the physician-patient chose to approach. Near the top of the agenda should be a frank inquiry as to how the patient feels being a patient and seeing this doctor. This can be done in a friendly and reassuring way but needs to be directly addressed.

It is wise to offer the physician-patient options—(remember, he just isn't prepared for the patient role)—that may include seeing another physician and seeking care in another clinic or city. The patient may be hesitant *not* to see a particular colleague as his physician for fear that he would offend if he sought care elsewhere.

The physician-patient's views, thoughts, observations must be heard and acknowledged. As a physician he may be a keen observer despite the other blocks to patienthood that he may experience and he may contribute considerable expertise to his care regarding his experience of his symptoms and illness. Similarly, the physician-patient's participation in particular discussions and decisions *in which any patient might participate* should be sought. Final decisions should generally be with the treating physician and attempts at self-care that have not been discussed must be confronted early. Stating the unequivocal need to discuss thoroughly any diagnostic or therapeutic options before they are undertaken will usually suffice and may be met with relief.

Difficult medical questions and tensions or difficulty in this therapeutic relationship may be aided by consultation from additional physicians. To excess, this can dilute and nullify what does need to be a potent and effective doctor-patient relationship. A "cast of thousands" is not a solution to problems that may arise with the physician-patient. Some consultation, however, is to be encouraged and can greatly increase the confidence and comfort of physician and patient alike. Consultation between the attending and a liaison psychiatrist may help the physician in dealing with his unique patient and gaining perspective on his therapeutic relationship.

If the physician-patient is hospitalized, it is the responsibility of the attending physician to acknowledge to the ward staff that this particular patient presents some complicated and unusual issues beyond that of most patients. If the issue is raised and the attending makes time available, nursing staff will usually ventilate, question, and discuss the care of this special patient with enthusiasm and appreciation.

The privacy and confidentiality of the physician-patient's care is important and should be discussed directly and early. If the patient does not raise questions in this regard, one can be almost certain that they do exist unspoken. Who will see the patient's chart? Who will be doing nursing procedures, tests, etc.? What information will be given out by the hospital regarding this stay? It is unwise to attempt to assure the patient absolute secrecy since this cannot usually be done and, if requested, probably reflects some undiscussed issues that the patient has about his illness and care. Reasonable privacy is crucial, however, and most visitors are probably best diverted, at least until the treatment program is understood and underway.

Physicians with illness, disability, or impairment, who do not willingly seek care, present special and even more complex problems. The literature dealing specifically with the impaired physician can be of help.[1,2]

County and state medical societies often offer aid and consultation regarding impaired colleagues. Many states have elaborate programs for confronting and dealing with the impaired physician that minimize disruption to him, his associates, and the care that he delivers to his patients. All physicians bear responsibility for recognition and action when ill colleagues do not seek care for themselves.

Finally, what can any physician do to avoid unnecessary personal impairment from stress or illness? Gorotivz[24] urges us to "step back from the daily grind" to assess our values, our leisure time, our life outside of our practices, and our ability to deal with the continuing and rapid changes in the medical care we deliver. As McCue[16] has stated, "It is unlikely that optimal medical care can be delivered by unhappy or maladjusted physicians . . .

Walking away from crises, refusing to acknowledge critical illness, and being unable to recognize one's insensitive or inadequate care are examples of denial found in impaired physicians." While we are unlikely ever to welcome the sick role ourselves, it is one of our most valuable professional and personal social conventions. It must, in fact, be protected and experienced to remain available. The learning that we as physicians may acquire in fully accepting and exploring the sick role ourselves can be some of the most valuable knowledge we can offer our patients.

Of all of the instruments we may use in the practice of medicine, our professional self is the most effective, the most valuable and, unfortunately, one of the most "neglectable." No CAT scanner, endoscope, or monitor would survive the level of care that many of us offer ourselves. We owe ourselves and our patients the best that we can deliver.

In caring for ill colleagues, we should remember that physicians are not intrinsically and inexplicably difficult and troublesome patients. The "difficult doctor" can be as much a part of the mystique and myth with which we have surrounded ourselves as reality. Rather, ill physicians are disconcerting to us and to themselves for understandable reasons based in who we are, what we've learned and experienced, and what we do for a living. The complicating factors can be recognized and addressed with benefit for all concerned.

REFERENCES

1. Arana GW: The impaired physician: A medical and social dilemma. *Gen Hosp Psychiatry* 1982; 4:147–154.
2. Sargent DA: The impaired physician movement: An interim report. *Hosp Comm Psychiatry* 1985; 36:294–297.
3. Von Brauchitsch H: The physician's suicide revisited. *J Nerv Ment Dis* 1976; 162:40–45.
4. Murray RM: Psychiatric illness in doctors. *Lancet* 1974; 1:1211–1213.
5. Vaillant GE, Brighton JR, McArthur C: Physicians use of mood-altering drugs: A 20-year follow-up report. *N Engl J Med* 1970; 282:365–372.

6. Murray RM: Alcoholism amongst male doctors in Scotland. *Lancet* 1976; 2:729–731.
7. Casterline RL: Deviant behavior in physicians. Read before the 69th Annual Congress on Medical Education of the American Medical Association, Chicago, February 9, 1973. As cited in Mawardi BH: Satisfactions, dissatisfactions, and causes of stress in medical practice. *J Am Med Assoc* 1979; 241:1483–1486.
8. Sharpe JC, Smith WW: Physician, heal thyself: Comparison of findings in periodic health examinations of physicians and executives. *J Amer Med Assoc* 1962; 182:234–237.
9. Robbins GE, MacDonald MC, Pack GT: Delay in the diagnosis of physicians with cancer. *Cancer* 1953; 6:624–626.
10. Hennekins C: Personal communication, 1985.
11. Talbott GD, Benson EB: Impaired physicians: The dilemma of identification. *Alcohol and Drug Problems* 1980; 68:56–64.
12. Vaillant GE, Sobowale NC, McArthur C: Some psychological vulnerabilities of physicians. *N Engl J Med* 1972; 287:372–375.
13. Duffy JC: *Emotional Issues in the Lives of Physicians.* Springfield, Ill, Charles C. Thomas, 1970.
14. McCue JD: The distress of internship. *N Engl J Med* 1985; 312:449–452.
15. Cousins N: Internship: Preparation or hazing? *J Amer Med Assoc* 1981; 245:377.
16. McCue JD: The effects of stress on physicians and their medical practice. *N Engl J Med* 1982; 306:458–463.
17. Edelstein EL, Baider L: Role reversal: When doctors become patients. *Psychiatria clinica* 1982; 15:177–183.
18. Seigler M, Osmond H: *Patienthood: The Art of Being A Responsible Patient.* New York, MacMillan, 1979.
19. Parsons T: *The Social System.* New York, Free Press, 1951.
20. Dlin BM: Masking the call for help: Encounters with colleagues in the corridor. *Psychosomatics* 1984; 25:25–29.
21. Stoudemire A, Rhoads JM: When the doctor needs a doctor: Special considerations for the physician-patient. *Ann Intern Med* 1983; 98:654–659.

22. Meissner WW, Wohlauer P: Treatment problems of the hospitalized physician. *Int J Psychoanalytic Psychotherapy* 1978–1979; 7:437–467.
23. Morse RM, Martin MA, Swenson WM, Niven RG: Prognosis of physicians treated for alcoholism and drug dependence. *J Amer Med Assoc* 1984; 251:743–746.
24. Gorovitz S: Preparing for the perils of practice. The Hastings Center Report, December 1984, pp. 38–41.

INDEX

Abdominal pain, 121, 126, 219, 228
Absence seizures, 163, 164
Achalasia, 123, 124
Aerophagia, 125
Alcohol
 abuse of in physicians, 271
 and depression, 235, 247
Alexander, Franz, 9–10
Alprazolam, 183
Alzheimer's disease, 258, 266
American Academy of Craniomandibular Disorders, 96
Amitriptyline, 68, 83, 117, 252
Aneurysm, 87, 88
Ankylosis, 96, 101–102
Anorexia nervosa
 age and sex distribution of, 20
 diagnosis of, 18–20
 DSM-III criteria for, 17–18
 family interactions in, 20–21, 25
 incidence of, 17, 20
 mortality rate in, 19
 treatment of, 21–26
  in hospital, 21–22
  medication, 24–25
  outpatient care, 25–26
  psychosocial, 22, 24
Antidepressants, 23, 25, 36–37, 53, 252–253
 in epilepsy, 244
 in fibromyalgia, 68–69
 in headache, 81
 in myofascial pain, 117
Antihistamines, 136, 199
Antipsychotics, 253
Anxiety, 127, 174–175, 214, 227, 228, 250–251
 anticipatory, 175, 181, 182, 183

Anxiety *(continued)*
case studies in, 250–251
causes of, 262–265
in conversion disorder, 223
diagnostic tests for, 265
differentiated from depression, 250
female preponderance in, 262
in somatization disorder, 214, 220
see also Panic attack
Anxiolytics, 23, 25, 53, 109, 183, 221
Arteritis, 87, 88
Arthritis; *see* Rheumatoid arthritis
Aspiration pneumonitis, 32, 34
Aspirin, 68, 100, 109, 247

Behavior modification, 23, 24, 109
Benzodiazepines, 101, 109, 183, 247
Bereavement, 232, 249–250
Binge eating; *see* Bulimia
Binge-purge cycle, 30, 36
Biofeedback, 81–82, 109–111, 129, 144, 148, 150–151, 155
Bipolar disorder, 237, 253, 266
Birth control pill; *see* Oral contraceptives
Body image, disturbance of, 18, 19
Borderline syndrome
characteristics of, 207
management of, 208
Brain, 214
Bruxism devices, 113
Bulimarexia; *see* Bulimia
Bulimia
complications of, 31–35
diagnosis of, 29–31
patient interview in, 30–31
DSM-III criteria for 29
incidence of, 28
treatment for, 35–37
behavioral, 35
medication, 36–37
psychotherapy, 36

Caffeine, 18, 83, 89, 133, 137, 180
Cardiac neurosis, 177
Cardiomyopathy, 18, 33, 34
Chest pain, atypical, 124–125, 176, 177, 178, 228, 262
Chronic pain syndrome, 60–61, 110; *see also* Pain, chronic
Colonic disorders, 125–128
treatment of, 128, 129
Constipation, 33, 35, 80, 121, 126, 127, 226, 267
Conversion disorder, 218, 223–225
age preponderance in, 223
differential diagnosis of, 224
treatment of, 225
Craniofacial pain, 87–88, 90, 96
Cushing's syndrome, 240, 248
Cyclothymic disorder, 231, 236

DaCosta, J. M. 177–178
Daily activity dairy, 145–146, 149
Dalton, Katherina, 52
Danocrine, 52
Defense mechanisms, 216–217
Degenerative joint disease, 98–99
Dementia, 242–243, 256–260
causes, 257

diagnostic tests for, 262
differential diagnosis of, 261
Depression, 231–253, 266–268
 in anorexia nervosa, 18, 25
 atypical, 236–237
 in bulimia, 30, 35, 36–37
 and cancer, 245–246, 266, 268
 and cardiovascular disease, 240–241
 case studies in, 232, 233, 234, 235–236, 237–238
 causes of, 266–269
 and central nervous system diseases, 242–245, 266, 268
 in chronic pain, 143, 148
 and diabetes, 240
 differential diagnosis of, 249–252
 drugs in, 238, 247–249, 266, 267
 and endocrine disorders, 238–240
 and epilepsy, 244
 in fibromyalgia, 65, 66, 67
 in headache, 71, 72, 76, 80, 86
 incidence of, 231
 in irritable bowel syndrome, 124, 127, 128–129
 masked, 227, 232
 with melancholia, 233
 in myofascial pain, 117
 and oral contraceptives, 46, 51, 248
 in premenstrual syndrome, 46
 with psychotic features, 233, 234–235, 237
 symptoms of, 219, 226–227, 232, 233, 235–236, 238
 tests for, 251–252, 268
 treatment of, 252–253
 and viral diseases, 241, 266
Dexamethasone suppression test, 251–252, 268
Diabetes, and depression, 240
Diagnostic and Statistical Manual, 3rd ed. (American Psychiatric Association) (*DSM-III*), 17–18, 29, 124, 231, 235, 236, 237
Diarrhea, 34, 35, 121, 126, 127, 129, 219, 228
Diazepam, 101, 109
Dieting, 20
Diuretics, 18, 22, 48, 53
Drugs
 abuse of
  in anorexia nervosa, 18, 19, 22
  in bulimia, 30, 34
  in physicians, 270–271, 277
 adverse reactions to
  in depression, 235, 247
  in panic attack, 180
 see also individual drugs
Duke Center for the Advanced Study of Epilepsy, 172
Dysthymic disorder, 231, 235–236

Eating disorders
 atypical, 17
 incidence of, 17
 see also Anorexia nervosa, Bulimia
Electroconvulsive therapy (ECT), 245–246, 253
EMG biofeedback; *see* Biofeedback
Endocrine disorders, 238–240
Epileptic seizures
 age distribution in, 163, 164, 166

Epileptic seizures *(continued)*
  and depression, 243
  differential diagnosis of, 163–167
    electroencephalography (EEG) in, 166, 264
  generalized, 162, 163, 166, 169, 172
  international classification of, 161–162
  partial, 163, 165–166, 168, 170, 172, 180, 181, 264
Escape behavior, 175
Esophagus
  disorders of, 121, 123–125
  treatment of, 129
Estrogen implants, 50, 51
Exercise, as therapy, 23, 49, 129
Eye, pain in, 73, 88

Factitial dermatoses
  case studies in
    malingering, 188–191
    pruritus, 197–199
    self-mutilation, 192–196
  evaluation of, 191
  patterns of, 188
Family therapy, 23, 24, 25, 36, 253
Fatigue, 18, 64, 74, 80, 81, 124, 219, 235, 242, 243, 262
Fever
  factitial, 203–208
    diagnosis of, 203–206
  low-grade, 208
  management of, 206–208
  psychiatric illness in, 206
  of unknown origin, 202–203, 204, 209
Fibromyalgia
  anatomical locations of, 59, 63
  case study, 58–59
  incidence of, 62
  personality traits in, 66–67, 68
  primary, criteria for, 62, 64
  secondary, 64
  therapy for, 68–69
Fibrositis; *see* Fibromyalgia

Ganser syndrome, 225–226
Gastric disorders, 121, 125
  treatment of, 129
Gonadotropin releasing hormone (GnRH), 51–52
Grief reactions, 214, 227, 249
Guilt
  in bulimia, 30, 33
  in depression, 232, 233, 243
  and headache, 80
Haloperidol, 197, 198, 245
Headache
  and allergy, 76
  and anxiety, 228, 262
  classification of, 77–79
  cluster, 73, 74, 82, 83, 85
  and depression, 71, 72, 80, 86, 232
  differential diagnosis of, 84
  exertional, 75, 86
  and hypertension, 73, 76, 85, 86
  and muscle tone, 80
  occupational, 75
  onset of, 71, 72, 75, 85
  precipitating factors in, 74–75
  psychogenic, 72, 78
  and sinuses, 72, 73, 85
  site of, 72, 80, 85
  and temporomandibular joint disorder, 96, 107
  in women, 72, 73, 76, 86, 89
  see also Migraine, Muscle contraction headache, Vascular headache

INDEX 287

Hearing disorders, 105, 219
Holmes, T. H., 215–216
Hydrocephalus, 244, 259
Hypercalcemia, 239, 267
Hyperthyroidism, 180, 239, 263
Hyperventilation, 177, 180–181
Hypochondriasis, 218, 222, 223
Hypoglycemia, 180, 181
Hypokalemia, 32, 33, 34, 35, 242, 266
Hypothyroidism, 239, 259
Hysterectomy, 50, 51

Imipramine, 36–37, 182, 251, 252
Influenza, and depression, 241
Intraoral appliances, 112
Ipecac syrup, 18, 32, 34
Irritable bowel syndrome
  anxiety in, 127–128
  depression in, 128–129
  examination for, 125, 127
    colonic, 125–126
    esophageal, 124
    gastric, 125
  incidence of, 120–121
  symptoms of, 121
  treatment for, 128–219

Joint disease, degenerative, 98–99

Lactate, in panic attack, 178
Lithium, 253
Locus ceruleus, 178, 240

Medroxyprogesterone acetate, 50, 51
Melancholia, 233, 241
Melatonin, 240

Menses
  cessation of in eating disorders, 19
  and headache, 80
  and somatization disorder, 219
  see also Premenstrual syndrome
Methylsurgide, 83
MHPG test, 251
Migraine, 72–75, 82–83
  classification of, 77–78
  ergotamine therapy for, 76, 83, 89
  as hereditary disorder, 75, 83, 85
  precipitating factors in, 74–75
  in pregnancy, 75
  prodrome, 73–74, 82
  and reserpine, 76
Mitral valve prolapse, 264
Monamine oxidase inhibitors, 182, 240, 248, 252
Mononucleosis, 208, 209, 241
Multiple sclerosis, 224, 245, 266
Munchausen syndrome, 226
Muscle contraction headache, 73, 76–77, 78, 80–82
  types of, 81
  treatment of, 81–82
Myoclonic jerks, 163–164
Myofascial pain, 96, 105–117
  treatment for, 107–117
Myotherapy, 113

National PMS Society, 54
Neurosyphilis, 241
Nonsteroidal anti-inflammatory agents, 68, 100, 108–109, 137, 247
Nutrition
  in eating disorders, 24
  in myofascial pain, 108
  in premenstrual syndrome, 47–49

Oral contraceptives
 and depression, 46, 51, 248
 and headache, 76, 89
 in premenstrual syndrome,
  45–46, 50–51
Organic affective syndrome, 238
Organic brain syndrome, 214,
 228
Osmond, H., 277
Osteoporosis, 52

Pain, chronic, 59, 68, 69, 81,
  138–156
 behaviors, 140
 case study, 138
 coping skills in, 142–145, 150–
  151
  behavioral, 143–144, 151
  cognitive, 142–143, 151
  psychophysiological, 144,
   151
 outpatient reinforcement in,
  156
 psychogenic, 225
 relapse prevention, 155–156
 testing in, 147
 treatment for, 139, 145–156
  activity recording, 145–
   146, 149
  behavorial, 139, 148
  building coping skills,
   150–155
  interviews, 145, 147
  medication monitoring,
   150, 153
Pain clinics, 139
Pain cycle, 140, 142, 143, 144,
 148
Pain Management Group, 150,
 151
Pain pathways, 66, 67–68

Pancreas, cancer of, 245–246,
 268
Panic attack, 174–183, 261
 age of onset, 177
 differential diagnosis of, 180–
  181
 female preponderance in, 177
 incidence of, 177
 symptoms of, 176–177, 178
 treatment of, 182–183
Parkinson's disease, 245, 249,
 258
Parsons, Talcott, 274
Pathophysiological problems
 and anxiety, 228
 depression and grief reactions,
  226–227
 factitious, 225–226
 and organic brain syndrome,
  228
 and schizophrenia, 228
 somatoform, 218–225
 symptom formation in, 213–
  218
Patienthood (Siegler & Osmond),
 277
Pellagra, 242
Pernicious anemia, 241–242,
 259–260
Pheochromocytoma, 86, 180,
 181, 264
Phobic behavior, 174, 183
Physicians
 characteristics of, 272–274
 and drug abuse, 270–271,
  277
 as patients, 274–279
PMS Action, 54
Polyuria, 35
Postejaculatory pain, 131, 135
Premenstrual Assessment Form,
 45

Premenstrual syndrome (PMS)
  counseling for, 53–54
  and depression, 240
  diagnosis of, 45–47
    psychological assessment, 46
  hormones in, 44, 50–52
  incidence of, 41
  symptoms of, 42–43
  treatment of, 47–54
Proctoscopy, 127
Progesterone, 44, 52, 53
Progressive muscle relaxation training, 144, 148
Propranolol, 81
Prostate
  cancer of, 132
  massage, 133, 136
Prostatitis
  bacterial, 131–132, 134, 135, 136
  definition of, 131
  nonbacterial, 132–133, 134, 135
Prostatodynia, 131–137
  clinical findings in, 135
  definition of, 132
  differential diagnosis of, 133–136
  and stress, 135, 136–137
  treatment of, 136–137
Pruritus, 197–199
Pseudodementia, 242–243, 260–261
Pseudoepileptic seizures, 166–172
  differential diagnosis of, 166–172
    age of onset, 169
    EEG in, 167, 168, 169, 172
    videotaping in, 168
  rage in, 169
  urinary incontinence in, 169, 170, 171
Psychogenic pain disorder, 218, 225
Psychotherapy
  in chronic pain, 148
  in depression, 253
  in eating disorders, 23, 24–26, 35–36
  in factitial syndromes, 196, 207–208
  in irritable bowel syndrome, 129
  in myofascial pain, 117
  for physicians, 272
Purpura, factitial, 188, 189
Pyridoxine, 48

Rahe, R. H., 215–216
Referred pain, 88
Reflux esophagitis, 124, 127
Reinforcement, 139–140
Reserpine
  in migraine, 76
  in depression, 267
Rheumatoid arthritis, 96, 99–101, 247
  therapy for, 100–101

Self-help groups, 23, 25–26
Self-infection, 205–206
Self-mutilation, 192–196
Serotonin, 66, 240, 245, 246, 267
Siegler, M., 277
Sleep disorders, 80, 226
  in depression, 232, 241, 243
  in fibromyalgia, 64, 65, 66
  in headache, 71
  in panic attack, 178
  in premenstrual syndrome, 49

Social Readjustment Rating
    Scale, 215–216
Somatization disorder, 218–221
    age of onset, 218
    differential diagnosis of, 219–220
    female preponderance in, 218
    treatment of, 220–221
Spironolactone, 53
Stimulants, 18, 35, 48, 248
Stress
    and conversion disorder, 224
    in excessive somatic concern,
        214–215
    and fibromyalgia, 66–67
    and headache, 74, 76
    and irritable bowel syndrome,
        121, 123, 124, 128–129
    and physicians, 272–273
    and prostatodynia, 135, 136–137
    in Social Readjustment Rating
        Scale, 215–216
Subarachnoid hemorrhage, 86, 88

Temporomandibular joint
    anatomy of, 91–94
    disorders
        diagnosis of, 97–98, 104,
            107, 112–113, 117
        female preponderance in,
            99, 107
        and hearing disorders,
            105
        symptoms of, 99, 104, 107
        treatment for, 100–101,
            102, 104, 107–109
    movement of, 94–96, 101
Tension headache; see Muscle
    contraction headache

Thermometer manipulation,
    204–205, 206
Tic douloureaux, 73, 79, 87–88
Transcutaneous electrical nerve
    stimulation (TENS), 110
Transurethral prostatectomy,
    136
Type A personalities, 123

Ulcers
    gastric, 125
    peptic, 121, 123, 125
Urination, 35, 135, 169, 170, 171

Valproic acid, 164
Vascular headache, 71–72, 78–79
    migraine type, 77
    nonmigraine type, 78, 83, 85
Visual disorders
    in headache, 73, 74, 82, 83, 87
    in somatization disorder, 219
Vitamin B_6, 44, 48, 51, 248
Vitamin B_{12}, 242
Vitamin deficiencies, 18, 248, 266
Vitamin E, 48–49, 86
Vomiting
    in conversion disorder, 219, 223
    in irritable bowel syndrome, 121
    in migraine, 74
    self-induced, 22, 29, 30
        complications of, 32–34

Weight loss, 18, 20, 21, 30, 34,
    126, 208, 226, 239, 240, 266